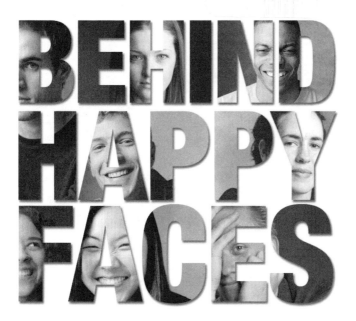

BEHIND HAPPY FACES

TAKING CHARGE OF YOUR MENTAL HEALTH

a guide for young adults

ROSS SZABO | MELANIE HALL

VOLT PRESS

11 10 09 08 07   5 4 3 2 1

Library of Congress Cataloging-in-Publication Data

Szabo, Ross.
  Behind happy faces: taking charge of your mental health, a guide for young adults / by Ross Szabo And Melanie Hall.
     p. cm.
  Includes bibliographical references.
  ISBN 978-1-56625-305-5 (pbk.)
  1. Mental health. I. Hall, Melanie (Melanie Whitley) II. Title.
  RA790.S975 2007
  616.89--dc22

                                    2007013703

VOLT PRESS (a division of Bonus Books, Inc.)
9255 W. Sunset Blvd., #711
Los Angeles, CA 90069
www.volt-press.com
www.bonusbooks.com

COVER DESIGN: *Candice Woo*
INTERIOR DESIGN: *Emily Brackett/Visible Logic*
ALL AUTHOR PHOTOS: *Cindy Gold*
FRONT COVER PHOTOS (L to R):
     Behind: *Ron Krisel/Ibid; Jim Newberry/Ibid; Marc L. Hauser/Ibid*
     Happy: *Ron Krisel/Ibid; Ron Krisel/Ibid*
     Faces: *Jim Newberry/Ibid; Ron Krisel/Ibid; Marta Garcia/Ibid*

Printed in the U.S.A.

Bonus Books/Volt Press titles may also be purchased at special **quantity discounts** for educational, business or promotional use. For more information please contact our Special Orders Department at (877) 660-1960 or specialorders@bonusbooks.com.

PRAISE FOR
Behind Happy Faces

"Ross Szabo has a true gift for getting through, and *Behind Happy Faces* allows him to communicate beyond the walls of a full school assembly. His book will most certainly reach you, and it will help you reach others. If it is understanding and compassion you seek, look no further."

—Lizzie Simon
Author, *DETOUR: My Bipolar Road Trip in 4-D*

"*Behind Happy Faces* removes the stigma surrounding mental disorders, and stimulates dialogue about these issues among high school and college students. Szabo and Hall are dynamic advocates for young people everywhere."

—Harold S. Koplewicz, M.D.
Chairman, Department of Child & Adolescent Psychiatry, NYU School of Medicine; Founder and Director, NYU Child Study Center

"Mental illness among young people is *epidemic*. Too often, those who are afflicted are ashamed, too often, they isolate themselves, and too often—the results are catastrophic. Frank, honest and informative, *Behind Happy Faces* will mitigate that shame and isolation, and so head off those dark results."

—Andrew Solomon
Author, *The Noonday Demon: An Atlas of Depression*

"An inspirational read for all young adults...as well as parents, teachers, family and friends, *Behind Happy Faces* provides tools for seeking help and gives hope for recovery. Ross is living proof that with treatment, young adults with mental health issues can be highly functional and lead fulfilling, productive lives."

—Tipper Gore
Photographer, Author and Mental Health Advocate

"Mental disorders *are* treatable and *don't* have to define one's life. *Behind Happy Faces* provides young people with an intimate glimpse into what it means to have an emotional disorder—and empowers them to overcome the stigma—to get the help they need."

—Donna Satow
Co-Founder, The Jed Foundation

"Szabo's enthralling narrative draws its strength from the power of his personal story, and the honesty with which he—and the other young people represented in the book—challenge the myths and stereotypes surrounding mental illness.

This powerful book deserves the WIDEST possible audience."

—Gail Griffith
Author, *Will's Choice: A Suicidal Teen, a Desperate Mother, and a Chronicle of Recovery*

*Vicky,
Embrace Your Freakishness!*

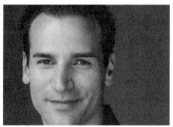

Ross E. Szabo (signature)

To my family—whose strength, love and unwavering support has made all the difference in my life.

—Ross

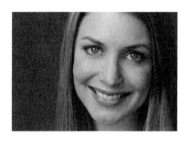

To my loving family.

—Melanie

CONTENTS

Chapter 5

THE "F" WORD:

Chapter 6

BEYOND YOUR BUDDY LIST:

PROLOGUE

Ross Szabo

High school was a really difficult time for me. Not only because of the usual stuff that most of us have to deal with, but mainly because bipolar disorder decided to enter my life the summer before my junior year. Things rapidly got worse, and in my senior year my depression became so severe that I had to be hospitalized. Two months after I got out of the hospital, a psychologist came into one of my classrooms and talked about some of the patients he was treating. Nearly every student in the room started laughing. After what I had been through myself, their laughter filled me with embarrassment and rage. Before I'd gone to that hospital, I was part of the "cool" crowd. I knew a lot of people and had a lot of friends. But things were totally different after I got out of the hospital. Suddenly I was the guy labeled with all of the negative stereotypes. I was the one people whispered about. I was the one who lost friends.

That day in class, I just couldn't take it anymore. I grabbed my teacher and pulled him out into the hallway. I told him I was upset, that I didn't think this was funny, and that it was pissing me off that people were laughing. He looked me square in the eyes and asked me what I wanted to do about it. I told him that *I* wanted to speak.

Two weeks later, I stood in front of that same classroom and spoke to the class about my *own* experiences related to my diagnosis of bipolar disorder, anger control problems, and psychotic features. I spoke from my gut. I was honest and open. And this time, *nobody laughed.* I didn't realize it at the time, but that day—in a basement classroom in Northampton Senior High School—was a major turning point for me.

That day marked the beginning of a lifelong journey for me, educating others about mental health issues. During the past five years as Director of Youth Outreach for the National Mental Health Awareness Campaign, I have had the opportunity to go to middle schools, high schools, and colleges all over this country, sharing my story and speaking about mental disorders. I've had the overwhelming experience of looking into the eyes of over 500,000 other young people. A lot of them also know what it's like to be laughed at—and have felt the pain related to all different sorts of common mental health problems.

After hearing from so many people over the years, it got to the point where each time I got up to speak, I was telling many of *their* stories. This is when I decided that I needed to write a book. I felt that I needed to take all of the similar things I kept hearing from so many young people and put them into writing, so that others could know that they are *not alone.* This book is the culmination of five years of tears, whispers, fear, and agony that I have seen on the faces of tens of thousands of people who are suffering. It's now time for everyone to move past the laughter—and really start *understanding* the common disorders that plague so many.

Melanie Hall

When my father was two years old, his dad placed a gun to his own temple and pulled the trigger. This bullet didn't just kill one man. It injured my whole family, inflicting damage as real as the wound that ended my grandfather's life.

My dad didn't learn the truth about his father's death until he was 11 years old, after a neighborhood boy taunted him during a game of kickball. "At least *my* dad didn't kill himself," the boy said.

This brief moment changed my dad's life forever. Many families often go out of their way to hide a suicide in their family history. They try to act as if it never happened, not realizing that the problems that caused the suicide in the first place can be passed on to each survivor. My family was different, and I thank both my mom and dad for having the strength to confront this reality and to teach me what it meant to deal with my own emotional issues. My parents refused to allow the legacy of my grandfather's death to continue in my life—or that of my sister's.

My grandmother always said that if my grandfather had lived a little longer, long enough to get help, then he would likely still be alive today. He had grown up during a time when it wasn't at all acceptable to even discuss one's mental health. Perhaps if he had been able to speak to someone, seek counseling, or even read a book like this to help him find the courage to work through his pain, things might have turned out differently.

Certainly it's a different time now, but you might be surprised to know that even despite the help that is now widely available, millions of people still continue to suffer in silence, fearing the consequences of confronting their issues. We *ALL* have problems. It's just part of being human. But whatever yours are, we hope that while reading this book, you come to realize that you're not the only one out there who's suffering—and that there's nothing to be ashamed of. But also know that each and every one of us is capable of getting help, tapping our strength, mustering our courage, and confronting our darkest secrets. But nothing will change if you keep pretending everything is okay, when in reality, you may need a little help. *It's up to you.*

INTRODUCTION

When people hear the word "mental," many of them will immediately think of the worst-case scenario. They think about things like depression. Or suicide. Or large-scale events like the tragic school shootings at Virginia Tech and Columbine. Or they may even conjure up images of wild-eyed people foaming at the mouth, wearing straitjackets, or carrying around axes in their cars. Sometimes they may think about the celebrities we're often seeing in the headlines who are continually exhibiting all kinds of erratic and out-of-control behaviors—impulsively shaving their heads, getting arrested for drunk driving, or checking into some form of "rehab" for everything from alcohol to homophobia.

But the overall issue of mental health doesn't just involve such extreme examples. Mental health is something every one of us should have—something each of us is entitled to. We all have emotional difficulties in our lives, and "mental health" simply means finding a way to handle those difficulties.

A "mental health issue" can refer to something as simple as dealing with stress about school, talking to someone you have a crush on for the first time, or worrying about your future. Further along the spectrum are life events that may be a bit more difficult to handle—things like your parents' divorce, the death of someone close to you, a relationship breakup, or the loss of a friendship. And then beyond that, there are more serious issues, things like anxiety disorders, clinical depression, and ADD/ADHD. Toward the extreme end of the spectrum are the most severe problems, including things like alcoholism, drug addiction, and mental disorders such as bipolar disorder, schizophrenia, eating disorders, and others.

If you think of mental health as an either/or thing—meaning, you're either out of your mind or you're not—it's hard to think about *changing* that state. But when you begin to think of mental health as a spectrum, it's much easier for you to determine exactly where you are on that spectrum, and what things you can do to move toward a healthier life.

Sadly, most young people never begin to explore this spectrum. The images surrounding the words "mental health" can be so negative and frightening that they are often afraid to even begin talking about many of their emotions. They may feel that people will judge them or label them in such a way that they will be considered outcasts. They buy into the common belief that anyone with a "mental" anything is assumed to be violent, scary, or so completely dysfunctional that they can't do anything like a "normal" person. But nothing could be further from the truth.

In today's culture, we have so many reasons to want to hide our true selves. There's a tremendous focus on appearances and huge pressure to be "the best." The fear of not being accepted, or not fitting in, has driven millions of people to hide the very thoughts, feelings, and emotions that are vital to their own individuality! There are a million reasons why you may feel the need to hide your pain. But if we're going to start taking mental health seriously, *the hiding needs to stop.*

Our hope is that this book will give you the courage to address those issues that have kept you from living the life you want, the courage to stop pretending that everything is OK (even when it's not), and more importantly, to stop hiding your true emotions...behind a happy face.

STARING INTO THE ABYSS:
The Facts About Mental Disorders

"Kids are different today
I hear every mother say..."
—Rolling Stones, "Mother's Little Helper"

ROSS' Story *One day when I was in the sixth grade, my dad came to pick me up from school. I climbed into the family minivan, and as we were driving down the highway, he turned to me and said that my oldest brother was in the hospital. At the time, my brother Thad was a sophomore at the University of Pennsylvania. I looked over at my dad to try to understand what he meant, and tears were streaming out from underneath his sunglasses.*

It was the first time I had ever seen my dad cry, so I asked him—was my brother hit by a car, did he break his leg, what happened? But my dad was so emotional he couldn't even speak. Later that night, my parents sat me down and told me that my brother wasn't only in the hospital, he was in the psychiatric ward. Now, I was just 11 years old. The only other time I had even heard of the "psychiatric ward" was in cartoons. I thought there was NO WAY my own brother could be in a place like that!

However, two weeks later, my parents, my middle brother and I all drove down to the University of Pennsylvania Hospital. I remember walking through security, seeing some people in straitjackets, and thinking to myself, there's NO way my brother is in here. But when we finally got to his door and saw him, I felt a little relieved. He didn't have an oxygen mask on his face, tubes in his arm, or casts on any part of his body. So of course I thought, he must be okay! But when I walked over to say hello to him, he didn't appear to know who I was. He didn't recognize my parents or my brother, either. He didn't even really understand that he was in a hospital.

On the way out of the hospital that day, everyone in my family was crying, except for me. My mom leaned down and told me it was all right if I wanted to cry. I then asked her if my brother was going to die, and she said no. So I told her that if he wasn't going to die, then I wasn't going to cry about it, because he must be able to get through this somehow.

I went on to watch my brother stay in the hospital for another two months. He took about a year off from college, but eventually returned. He ultimately graduated from Penn with a degree in physics, then went on to Florida State University and got his master's in physics. Today, he is in the process of getting his doctorate in Astrophysics at the University of Southern California. So, maybe my brother is a bit of a freak—(I have a hard time understanding math, let alone physics!)—but the point is, he is an example of someone who has managed to deal with his mental disorder really well, and set his life back on a positive track.

Why Do I Need to Worry About Mental Health?

When you hear the words "mental health," you may not even fully understand what they mean. Some think the term is only referring to people with mental disorders—depression, anorexia, schizophrenia. Others assume that mental health is something you should only be concerned about if you have a major emotional issue to deal with—a divorce, a breakup, the death of someone you love. But the reality is that mental health is an important issue for everyone. Each one of us needs to find a way to deal with the problems we're experiencing, no matter how big or small they may seem. Finding productive ways to do that is what mental health is all about.

High school and college are stressful times for everybody. There's no escaping it. Growing up can feel like a ride on a roller coaster. Your moods can change faster than the speed of sound. Huge decisions are hanging over your head. What college should you apply to? What major should you choose? Who should you be dating? Should you be hooking up with someone? To some extent, all of this is normal. When you're struggling to figure out who you are and what you want to do with your life, sometimes it doesn't take much to make you feel totally out of control. "Keep up your grades. Play a sport—or two. Learn an instrument. Get involved in every extra-curricular activity possible. Volunteer for any and every cause under the sun. It will look better on your college application..." Sound familiar? If you haven't already noticed, the competition to be accepted at a good college is fierce these days, and has only intensified over the years. In 2005, nearly half (47%) of college freshmen had an A average in high school, compared with 20% of freshmen in 1970. Once you get to college, the pressure doesn't fade. You have to worry about your GPA. You need to figure out what you're going to do when you finish school. You need to arrange for that internship this summer and build up your life experience.

With all this going on, is it at all surprising to you that the number one mental health issue facing college and high school students today is simply...*lack of sleep?* That's right. If you've ever been awake for 24 hours or more at a stretch, you know how functional you are by that point—not very. An extremely effective way to break a person down is to only allow him or her sleep three to five hours a night. A lot of college students report sleeping between only four and six hours. And while experts agree that most high school students ideally need nine to 10 hours of sleep, most studies show they are averaging less than seven. When you're sleeping that little, you're bound to be stressed out.

And stress can come from plenty of places outside of yourself. For example, there's nothing like having the rug ripped

Our Brains Need Interaction!

We know that the breakdown of the family can make it hard for kids to trust or feel close to others. But one particular study went even further. A group of researchers was interested in what was happening to the development of children's brains in today's age of family separation. The study took neuro-images (MRIs) of the brains of four-year-olds in African hunter-gatherer tribes, and neuro-images (MRI's) of the brains of four-year-old American children. They found that the brains of the children in the tribes were larger, more fully connected, and more fully developed. Human brains are wired to grow through touch and interaction, and while there is a ratio of 25 to 30 adults for each child in a tribe, it is hard to find even a single adult for each child in America.

out from under you when suddenly your parents announce their divorce. The national divorce rate is close to 50% these days, so I know many of you are having to deal with this situation in your own family. And even if your parents stay together, that doesn't guarantee a stress-free ride. In most families today, both parents work. If you were raised in such a family, you probably had limited interaction with your parents—or maybe you had to take on other responsibilities to help out. Not feeling connected with your family is tough, and it can make it even harder to deal with other problems that life throws your way.

Coping Mechanisms:
Why Some Are Better Than Others

Maybe a *lack* of family interaction isn't your problem. Some people are shadowed by an overly attentive mom or dad—otherwise known as the "helicopter parent." It's the mom who calls between every class or picks her son's subjects at school. It's the dad who regularly talks to his daughter's professors, does all her laundry, knows all her friends. These parents are protecting their children from having to live their own lives, having to take responsibility for their own choices. When a parent acts too much as a shelter, the children never learn to develop their own ways of coping with things. For a time, they may not feel life's stressors as much as their peers do, but it's only a matter of time. The parent cannot be there to protect them forever. And when the reality of life hits someone for the first time as an adult, it can be even harder to deal with.

But you can't go and live in a cave. There's no avoiding these kinds of stress. Your only choice is in how you deal with them. And truth be told, many of our coping mechanisms, well…they suck.

"There must be a way out," you think. An easier way to deal. Something, *anything.* But there isn't, so when you have time, you try to escape. You text or instant message your friends, or post on their profiles. You communicate constantly, but for the most part, you're really saying less. When you do have emotional problems, communicating online limits you to a "crying" emoticon, instead of *actually* crying in front of someone who cares about you. That is, if you ever allow yourself to cry at all.

Some cry to relieve stress, while others *shop*. It's practically become a religion to many of us these days. Exposure to the media makes it hard to avoid the message that you can *spend* your way to happiness. The average woman sees 400 to 600 advertisements per day, telling her how she could be a complete and happier person, *if only* she would buy this new product! All of these commercials can be totally overwhelming. It's almost like we're all being brainwashed.

Or you may think, isn't it easier to deal – by just *not* dealing, by numbing out to your favorite drug? Maybe. You may look around and see your friends popping pills, or maybe even their friends' pills. Whether it's Ritalin to study, a Xanax to chill, or an anti-depressant of some kind, maybe you're just searching for a quick fix. Unfortunately, a "quick fix" doesn't do much to help with deep-seated, ongoing emotional problems.

Those of you searching for relief from the pressure may have tried various methods—some more productive than others—like overdoing it on the double lattes, exercising too much, playing a sport, writing, or just doing something creative. But many of us decide to go for broke instead. We take things too far and go out and "party" or get smashed, hammered, tipsy, crunk, high, wasted—anything to try to relieve all the pressures that have built up. Pressures we're choosing not to deal with in healthier, more effective ways.

While the rates of people using marijuana, cocaine, heroin, and some other hard-core drugs have slightly declined, the abuse of crystal meth and prescription drugs is still high. In fact, a lot of people aren't even trying to get a prescription. Why bother? They don't have to. The pills are everywhere. They can just float a few from a friend.

Did You Know?

Over 44% of college students report binge drinking, and two-thirds of young people with a substance use disorder *also* have another mental health issue.

Partying isn't the only way to have a good time or "take the edge off."

Whether it's "friends with benefits," a one-night stand, or being in an exclusive relationship, an estimated 80% of college students and 47% of high school students are sexually active. Maybe you think, why even bother going to college if you're never going to hook up with anyone? It's part of the campus culture. Or you feel a lot of pressure, worried you may be the last virgin in high school (trust us, you're *not*). This isn't necessarily a suggestion to cruise around school with your chastity belt locked—everyone has to choose for themselves if and when they are ready for sexual intercourse. But be careful, as sex can also be dangerous if it's used like a drug in an attempt to numb your emotions or hide from major life problems.

Sex, drugs, or even too much exercise or a quick shopping trip to the mall—any of these can be used to temporarily distract yourself from your emotional pain. Sometimes it even becomes a competition. For some, it's almost a badge of honor to be the one who can sleep less, drink more, handle the most stress, deal with the largest problems—but this is a game that no one wins.

You can choose to stay quiet about what hurts you—or worse, you can go numb while you just assimilate into a culture that regularly encourages you to disassociate from your feelings. *Drink* more. *Buy* more. Have *sex* with more partners. Keep *hiding* behind a happy face, a fake smile— pretending that everything's okay. Do anything but feel the truth of your reality.

Not So Sexy

According to Health Services at Columbia University, 25% of college students have a sexually transmitted illness (STI). The U.S. Center for Disease Control and Prevention reports that two-thirds of all people with an STI are under the age of 25, and 80% of them don't even realize they have one.

We all face a good deal of stress and pressures in our daily lives, but should we be terrified about the kind of world we're living in? No. These things need to be pointed out because they're real and you need to understand the problems to be able to find the solutions. There *are* healthier ways to deal with things. You can talk about these issues with a friend, family member, counselor, or anyone you feel you can trust. Chances are, you'll learn that some of these other people are in the same boat, and simply allowing yourself to talk about it can actually help to release some of your stress. But in order to learn to talk about your feelings, you need to first get over the fear or the mindset that "everyone's going through their own issues, so I'm just going to stay silent." It's really *okay* to share. It's *okay* to talk. In fact, talking is one of the healthiest things you can do for yourself!

What are some others? You can develop friendships that aren't based on drinking, drugs or doing other destructive things together. You can try to find ways to adjust your daily routine so that it leaves you more time to get enough sleep. If you are doing anything negative or destructive in an effort to cope with the stress in your life, identify it and try to find a way to replace it with something healthy. As you read on, you will find a lot of tips throughout this book that can help you with this.

What is a Mental Disorder?

But what if what you're feeling isn't just ordinary stress? What if it's something more intense, something that's scaring you? Now we're talking about a new place on the mental health spectrum—mental *disorders*. A mental disorder is a great deal more severe than just the everyday stress of life. The easiest definition is a pronounced shift in mood, thoughts, or functioning that lasts for two or three weeks or more that makes it impossible for someone to do the things he or she typically does.

A mental disorder is not just having about "good days" or "bad days." It's not just about going through a death, divorce, or breakup situation either. Usually when someone has a diagnosable mental disorder, they don't have a clearly identifiable cause for the way they're feeling. It is possible for a traumatic life event to trigger a mental disorder, but once someone is afflicted with any disorder, he or she may feel like *everything* in their life is going wrong, not just one particular thing. The good news is that all of these disorders are much more diagnosable—and *treatable*—today than ever before, especially if you seek help early.

If you have a history of mental disorders in your family, then you are more at risk for developing one yourself. But these disorders can also come from a negative environment and can be triggered even if there is *no* family history. To help you recognize those moments when what you're feeling might be something more than just everyday stress or anxiety, we've listed the most common disorders below, as defined by the National Institute of Mental Health. Read each description carefully and see if anything strikes a chord with you.

Remember, life is all about ups and downs. Everyone has his good days and his bad days, but when your ups and downs are *so* extreme that they disable you—keeping you from functioning normally for more than a period of two or three weeks—then you need to visit a mental health professional. It's possible you could have a mental disorder.

Common Mental Disorders: Descriptions and Symptoms

Anxiety Disorders are the most common mental disorders, affecting over 40 million American adults each year. Anxiety is a normal reaction to stress and helps people deal with difficult situations such as studying for tests, delivering a presentation, or dealing with a roommate. But when anxiety becomes an excessive, irrational fear of everyday situations, it can become disabling. Anxiety disorders can make you feel as though you are having a heart attack—like the walls are caving in, you can't breathe, you're going to die—you feel like you can't escape the fear. Anxiety attacks can come from a lot of different sources, and attempts to calm the anxiety can actually result in someone having multiple disorders. The most common anxiety disorders are generalized anxiety disorder, obsessive-compulsive disorder, panic disorder, post-traumatic stress disorder, and social anxiety disorder.

Depression, also called clinical depression, is the second most common mental disorder. Its symptoms are persistent sad, anxious, or "empty" moods; sleeping too much or too little; dramatic changes in appetite and/or weight; loss of pleasure and interest in activities you once enjoyed, including sex; restlessness, irritability; difficulty concentrating, remembering, or making decisions; fatigue or loss of energy; feeling guilty, hopeless or worthless; and even thoughts of suicide or death.

Eating disorders are the third most common mental disorders. The three main types of eating disorders are *anorexia, bulimia* and *binge-eating disorder.*

- **Anorexia** shows up as extreme weight loss and a belief that you are fat, despite excessive thinness. Symptoms can include frequently skipping meals, taking tiny or insufficient portions, not eating in front of others, always finding an excuse not to eat, hair loss, looking pale or malnourished, detesting all or specific parts of your body, insisting that you cannot feel good about yourself unless you're thin, and becoming socially isolated by withdrawing into yourself.

- **Bulimia** means regularly binge-eating and then attempting to prevent weight gain by immediately purging (vomiting, abusing laxatives, exercising excessively). Some common signs of bulimia include frequent binging, usually in secret; buying "binge food" (usually junk food or food high in calories, carbohydrates and sugar); unusually excessive dental problems (acid from purging can cause tooth enamel to erode), leaving clues that suggest you really want someone to realize what is going on (empty food packages, foul-smelling bathrooms, running water to cover sounds of vomiting, use of breath fresheners, poorly hidden containers of vomit); and using laxatives, diet pills, water pills or "natural" products excessively to promote weight loss.

- **Binge eating disorder** refers to frequent episodes of binge eating (eating a huge amount of food in a short period of time, while feeling that you don't have control over what you're eating). In a binge-eating episode, at least three of the following descriptions will usually ring true: you eat much more rapidly than normal; you eat until you feel uncomfortably full; you eat large amounts of food even though you're not really hungry; you eat alone because you feel embarrassed by how much you're eating; you feel disgusted with yourself, depressed, or very guilty after overeating. Binge eating occurs, on average, for two days a week for six months. The binging is similar to bulimia, except that if you have binge eating disorder, you don't actually purge the food from your body, which typically causes you to be overweight for your age and height.

Attention Deficit Disorder/Attention Deficit Hyperactivity Disorder, also known as ADD or ADHD, is the fourth most common mental disorder in college students. These disorders can make it hard to function at home, at school, and in relationships with friends. You act impulsively, you can't sit still, you talk while others are talking, or you're constantly daydreaming and unable to pay attention.

Bipolar Disorder is also known as *manic depression* and affects more than two million Americans each year. Along with symptoms of depression, people living with bipolar disorder also exhibit symptoms of mania: excessive energy, activity, restlessness, racing thoughts, and rapid talking. You might deny that anything is wrong and feel an extreme "high" or euphoria. Other signs include being easily irritated or distracted; not sleeping much, or at all; feeling extremely confident or optimistic; showing poor judgment; possessing unusual sexual drive; abusing drugs, particularly cocaine, alcohol or sleeping medications; behaving in provocative, intrusive, or aggressive ways; and sometimes even having delusions or hallucinations.

Schizophrenia is a chronic, severe, and disabling brain disorder that affects about one percent of people around the world. If you have schizophrenia, you may sometimes hear voices that others can't, believe that others are broadcasting their thoughts to the world, or become convinced that people are plotting to harm you. This can make you fearful and withdrawn, making it difficult when you try to have relationships with others.

Borderline Personality Disorder (BPD) affects about 2% of adults, mostly young women. If you have it, your moods, relationships, feelings about yourself, and behavior change constantly, disrupting nearly every part of your life. Symptoms include intense bouts of anger, depression and anxiety that may last for a period of hours or even a full day. With BPD, your social relationships are almost never stable. Your attachments to others may be intense but stormy, and your attitudes towards family, friends, and loved ones may suddenly shift—from great admiration and love, to intense anger and dislike whenever a slight separation or conflict occurs. BPD often occurs in conjunction with other psychiatric problems, particularly bipolar disorder, depression, anxiety disorders, substance abuse, and other personality disorders.

While these next two aren't technically mental disorders, they can inhibit people just as much:

Substance Abuse refers to the addiction to, or abuse of, drugs or alcohol. There are many symptoms and warning signs: you use the substance on a regular basis (daily, weekends or in binges); you develop a tolerance for it; you try to stop using it but can't; if you stop using the substance, you have physical withdrawal symptoms (trembling, hallucinations, sweating, high blood pressure), and in some cases, dementia.

Self-injury is also called *self-mutilation, self-harm,* or *self-abuse.* It means hurting yourself deliberately, repetitively, impulsively, but in ways that don't lead to death. Some examples of self-injury can include cutting, scratching, picking scabs or interfering with wound healing, burning, punching yourself or other objects, infecting yourself, inserting objects in your body openings, bruising yourself or breaking bones, some forms of hair-pulling, as well as other various forms of bodily harm. Possible warning signs include unexplained frequent injuries including cuts and burns, and always wearing long pants and long sleeves (even in warm weather). But the signs of self-injury can also be more subtle, like low self-esteem; difficulty handling feelings; relationship problems; and doing poorly at work, school, or home.

You Are Not Alone

Mental disorders can be disabling, life-altering, and when you're in the midst of one—completely consuming. They control your thoughts, destroy your ability to function, and threaten your hopes for the future. These disorders can lead to dropping out of school; losing friendships or relationships; or not being able to work, study, or do the things you once enjoyed. And, in the worst case, mental disorders can even lead to death. But it doesn't have to be this way. If you think you have a disorder, you *can* get help. That's one of the things you will learn from reading this book.

Most of us know at least one person who has been touched by a mental disorder. Maybe it's a friend or family member who has the disorder, or maybe *you* are the person suffering. Oftentimes, we have have no clue what to say or do about it. This book will show you what it's like to suffer from these disorders, and provide you with options for what you can do if you know someone who does. But most importantly, this book will give you *hope*. You'll learn tips on how to survive the storm. You'll hear firsthand accounts of what you can do for yourself, how to deal with a friend, what you can do in a family situation, and how to manage relationships while going through a mental disorder.

In each chapter, you'll meet people who have not only dealt with some of the most difficult mental disorders, but who have also found a way to move forward with their lives in a positive way – while also helping others.

We hear complaints every day that there's no way to deal with these disorders, but we disagree. We *know* there is hope. There is indeed a light at the end of the tunnel (and no, it's not a locomotive speeding towards you!). Statistics show that a large majority of people who seek help can see improvement in their symptoms. They can go back to functioning the way they used to. However, the key to resuming your life is getting the help you need, when you need it. In order to get well, *you must ask for help.*

Mental disorders are difficult, but they don't have to be a death sentence. That may have been true for some in the past, but it isn't anymore. We have learned more about the brain just over the past 10 years than we ever knew in the previous two thousand. It's time to *remove the stigma* around terms like "mental health" or "mental illness" or "mental disorders" that keeps so many people from talking about this issue. It's time to stop hiding behind our happy faces, and start taking care of ourselves—and each other.

Some Truths About Mental Disorders

- Suicide is the third leading cause of death in high school students and the second leading cause of death in college students.[1]

(more)

Some Truths About Mental Disorders (cont.)

- Over 66% of young people with a substance use disorder also have another mental health issue.[2]

- 19% of high school students report seriously considering attempting suicide, 14.8% make a specific plan, and 8.8% actually attempt it.[3]

- 12 million children and adolescents suffer from a diagnosable form of a psychiatric disorder. [4]

- Serious emotional disturbances affect one in every ten young people, but an estimated two-thirds are not getting the help they need.[5]

- 50% of mental illness begins by adolescence and often gets worse later in life.[6]

- The most common mental disorders are anxiety disorders, followed by depression (including bipolar disorder), eating disorders, ADD/ADHD, schizophrenia and borderline personality disorder.[6]

- In 2005, 90.3% of college counseling centers reported a rise in students with severe psychological problems, and 95% reported a rise in students who were already on psychiatric medications going to counseling centers.[7]

- The freshman year of college is the most "at-risk" year. Freshmen die at a higher rate from illness than other students, they account for 40% of undergraduate deaths from natural causes, and they account for 40% of undergraduate suicides.[8]

- 10% of college students report having suicidal thoughts; 45% report depression.[9]

- 40% of college men and 50% of college women surveyed said they had suffered depression so severe at some point that they could barely function; 14.9% said they had actually been diagnosed with depression; over 60% reported "feeling things were hopeless" one or more times during previous years; 95% report feeling "overwhelmed" at times.[10]

- Students are abusing psychiatric medications not prescribed to them. 14% of students at a midwestern liberal arts college reported borrowing or buying prescription stimulants from each other, and 44% knew someone who had done so.[11]

- Eating disorders occur most frequently in college-age women.[12]

1. National Mental Health Association; 2. Surgeon General's Report on Suicide and Mental Health (1999); 3. Youth Risk Survey (2001); 4. New York University Child Study Center; 5. New York University Child Study Center; 6. National Institute of Mental Health; 7. National Survey of Counseling Center Directors (2005); 8. USA Today (January 25, 2006); 9. College of the Overwhelmed, Dr. Richard Kadison (Jossey-Bass, 2005); 10. American College Health Association (2004); 11.The Journal of American College Health; 12. American Psychiatric Association

CHAPTER 2

THERE'S NOTHING WRONG WITH ME:

The Reasons We Hide

"I'm not crazy, I'm just a little unwell,
I know right now you can't tell."
—Matchbox 20, "Unwell"

ROSS *At age 16, I started to experience the symptoms of bipolar disorder. It first started with sudden and extreme mood swings. I wouldn't be able to sleep for like four days at a time, and I wouldn't sleep for more than an hour a night for up to two weeks at a time. I would go to school, play basketball, party and feel on top of the world. But then my moods* *would change. I would get really angry and violent, punching and kicking things, and I'd totally flip out on my parents and friends. Then my moods would change again, to where I couldn't even bring myself to get out of bed.*

Because my mind was going through so much, I felt like I just wanted to shut it down. And the quickest way I knew to shut my mind down was to drink. At age 16, I would drink a case of beer and pass out—drink a bottle of rum and pass out—drink a bottle of vodka and pass out.

When I was in high school, we had to listen to presentations where speakers would come in and tell us, "DON'T DRINK... because alcohol is bad for you." Well, I can tell you there was never really a day when I woke up hung over or puking my guts out when I thought alcohol was actually good for me, so I didn't really need someone to tell me that. But the thing is, no one ever came into my school and said, "Hey Ross – DON'T DRINK just because you hate yourself," or "DON'T DRINK as an escape because you don't know how to talk about your problems," or "DON'T DRINK because you can't come up with a better way of dealing with things..."

Luckily, my middle brother Vance told a friend of the family about everything I was going through, and our friend suggested I visit a psychiatrist. I went to see one soon after, explained my symptoms for like two hours, and I was diagnosed with bipolar disorder. I wish the story could stop here. But much like the first diagnosis of many problems, this was actually just the tip of the iceberg.

At age 17, my diagnosis evolved to include "bipolar disorder with anger control problems and psychotic features." During

BehindHappyFaces.com

the summer before my senior year of high school I started having extreme outbursts of anger. I actually broke some of my knuckles and toes from punching and kicking things. I even started having severe hallucinations of people chasing me, and I was hearing voices that were telling me to kill myself, or my friends. As you might imagine, all of these extreme changes caused me to later plunge into a deep depression during my senior year.

That same year, I was ultimately hospitalized for wanting to take my own life. But you should know that what led me there didn't all just happen in one day, for any one particular reason. In September, I started experiencing increasing feelings of loneliness. But I didn't talk to anyone about it, I guess because I thought that was a sign of weakness. I really thought that one day, I would wake up and those feelings would go away. But...they didn't.

It was November when I then started having thoughts of death, thoughts of suicide. That soon escalated to the point where I was thinking about death and suicide nearly 24 hours a day, seven days a week. But as frightened as I was, I still hadn't told anyone about it. For two solid months of my senior year, it seemed like anytime I was by myself I was crying—but whenever I was in front of people, I would just strut around school like always, smiling as though nothing was wrong, nothing out of the ordinary. I laughed with other people. Talked about the things everyone else was talking about. I just made a habit of sacrificing my own true thoughts and emotions for the sake of everyone else. But at the time, I was honestly convinced that one day I would just wake up, my personal nightmare would *be over, and I would want to live again. Unfortunately, that day never came.*

Why Is It So Hard to Seek Help?

Ross suffered for a long time without seeking help, partly because he was afraid of being perceived as weak, gutless, overemotional, a wuss, a wimp. Have you ever felt this way? The fact is, a whopping 66% percent of young people with a mental disorder *don't* seek the help they need. Let's explore some of the various reasons why—you may be able to identify with one or more of them.

"People Will Think I'm Crazy"

No one wants to be thought of as "crazy." It's a social cancer, a stigma, a straitjacket of a judgment that's hard to remove once you've been made to wear it. "Crazy" is an antiquated term that gets applied to people whenever they deviate from the "norm." In 2005, when comedian Dave Chapelle stunned both fans and the entertainment industry by abruptly leaving the country in the midst of production of his TV series *Chapelle's Show*, many in the press were quick to brand him as having gone "crazy." Chappelle later claimed that he had merely taken a leave for his own personal reasons, and that the harsh mistreatment by the press left him feeling misunderstood and dehumanized. This is very often the case when someone is thoughtlessly written off as being "crazy." Who the person is, and what he stands for—ends up being dismissed, forgotten. In turn, the accused "crazy" person often takes this as a sign that maybe there *is* something irreparably wrong with him. He then turns society's stigma against himself. The result? He starts having feelings of worthlessness, guilt, anger, confusion, fear, and a whole host of other negative emotions.

A Safe Place

FacetheIssue.com is a website that was created to give young people a safe place where they could talk about their problems and find mutual support—*anonymously*. There was clearly a need for such a place, as within 24 hours of launching the campaign, over 300,000 people had visited the site! The message boards were quickly filled with heart-wrenching stories about eating disorders, domestic abuse, sexual abuse, self-mutilation, depression, and many other unimaginably painful issues. For some of those first visitors, it was the first time they had ever openly shared their emotions and fears with anyone. When you visit the site, you will also discover several very cool animated videos, narrated by A-list celebs (Jennifer Lopez, Sarah Jessica Parker, Kate Hudson, Nicole Kidman, etc.) who wanted to do their part to help young adults feel more comfortable about facing these common emotional issues.

Just what *is* "crazy" supposed to mean, anyway? Well, according to Merriam-Webster's Dictionary, the word **crazy** is defined as:

> *1a: full of cracks or flaws : UNSOUND b : CROOKED, ASKEW*
>
> *2a: MAD, INSANE b (1) : IMPRACTICAL (2) : ERRATIC c : being out of the ordinary : UNUSUAL <a taste for crazy hats>*
>
> *3a: distracted with desire or excitement <a thrill-crazy mob> b: absurdly fond : INFATUATED <he's crazy about the girl> c: passionately preoccupied : OBSESSED*

Do you know a single person who's never been "impractical," "erratic," "unusual," "infatuated," or "obsessed?" If you're engaged in life and have emotions (which, by the way, we ALL do) then by definition—chances are, even *you* may wear the "crazy" badge once in a while. Especially when you're young, and still trying to figure so many things out. But if you choose to let the fear of being called "crazy" keep you from being honest with yourself and talking about your problems, you're just setting yourself up for even more trouble.

ANNABELLE had been diagnosed with clinical depression. But other than her own parents, she hadn't told a soul. *I'm sort of scared I'll be thought of as a "psycho"* *or something if I tell anyone about it. But it's upsetting—I constantly think about death—I'll imagine my own funeral, or the funerals of everyone close to me. Most nights I either cry myself to sleep, or I hardly sleep at all. And no matter what I do, it's like I can't stop thinking about it. Which also makes it impossible for me to really enjoy anything the way I used to. These thoughts have been running through my head for so long now, but I've just tried to keep them to myself. I guess because I'm afraid of what they mean, or what people may think if I try to talk about it.*

Another problem for Annabelle was that her family didn't fully understand depression. They didn't know what to do with this news of her diagnosis. More importantly, they shared many of Annabelle's same fears and anxieties about what her diagnosis meant, and how she—or *they*—might be perceived if anyone were to find out about it. So instead of learning more about her disorder, her family shut down, went into denial, almost trying to pretend it wasn't really happening, while Annabelle just fell into an even deeper depression.

A diagnosis like depression is often misunderstood, but it's also extremely common. In fact, it's the second most frequently diagnosed mental disorder in the country. But unfortunately, there is a prevailing message in our culture that says if you have depression, or any other sort of mental disorder, then something must be severely wrong with you. You're different. Weird. Maybe even *crazy*. And that whatever you do—you certainly shouldn't let anyone else know about it.

MARTHA's mother has schizophrenia and her father suffers from alcoholism. At age 11, Martha realized she was having some problems of her own.** *Nothing seemed to make me feel happy anymore—everything just seemed to make me sad. I began to think that something was seriously wrong with me, which was scary because I didn't know why this was happening, or if it would ever go away.*

I had never felt comfortable going to speak with the school guidance counselor about anything, because mostly it seemed that just those kids with special needs or behavioral problems went to the counselor's office, and I didn't want to be lumped in with those kids. I didn't want to be like my mom. I didn't want people to start calling me "crazy." And I didn't want anyone to think that there was something wrong with me. I was afraid my teachers or my classmates would just think I was weak or that I couldn't handle myself.

Eventually I ended up calling a suicide hotline. Not because I really wanted to take my own life, but more because I just felt that I had to talk to someone. But then I felt so humiliated and embarrassed for even needing to make the call that I just hung up the phone as soon as they answered.

Oftentimes, people treat the notion of a mental disorder as something that can never really be changed, like a Scarlet

Letter you'll have to wear for the rest of your life. It seems like everywhere you turn, the examples we're always seeing of people being associated with the concept of mental illness or mental disorders are *extreme* ones (violent criminals, serial killers—people who are completely dysfunctional). But in reality, most people with mental disorders are not like that at all. And it seems you rarely hear about all the positive stories of so many people out there—people with depression, bipolar disorder, alcoholism—who have found treatment, learned to deal with their issues, and who now lead a normal life.

When you grow up with no positive examples of people with mental disorders, fearing that people will wrongly judge you if you admit to having any of these types of issues, it's easy to want to give up. Sometimes it's just too hard to imagine that life could actually improve. But one point this book will continue to stress is that a mental disorder does *not* have to define your life. These disorders are treatable. *There is hope.*

The negative stereotypes out there can be very overwhelming—especially if you're just starting to realize that you may have a mental disorder. Don't forget that while the people you'll read about in this book have endured some traumatic situations, they have also managed to find the tools to cope with their lives in a healthy way. They are living proof that you don't have to fear the judgment of the rest of the world. You can have a diagnosis like bipolar disorder and still be a highly functional, happy person. It's okay. You don't need to be afraid anymore.

"It's Not That Big of a Deal"

When you stop and think about the intensity of human suffering we've witnessed as a society in recent years, it's easy to feel as if your own personal problems pale in comparison. Unthinkable traumatic events like September 11th, the war in Iraq, Hurricane Katrina, the tsunami in Asia, genocide in Darfur, and the African AIDS crisis can make anyone's day-to-day issues seem rather trivial sometimes, if not completely unimportant. Catastrophic world events can make it easy for anyone to try to minimize his or her problems—but so can larger personal tragedies. This causes many people to make light of their issues and their feelings, failing to realize the extent to which they need help.

COLLEEN was 14 years old when she was first diagnosed with anxiety, depression, and an eating disorder. *I suppose that in my teens, when things got serious, I didn't try to seek help at first because I didn't totally realize that I needed it. I tended to put my mental health on the back burner because it just always seemed too hard to handle and too inconvenient.*

If you postpone or neglect dealing with your mental health, some disorders have the power to evolve quickly and severely, overwhelming your capacity to cope or fully understand what is happening to you. Like a light rainstorm that suddenly morphs into a category five hurricane, the first initial symptoms can seem as minor as a rainy day. Let's use an anxiety disorder as an example. It starts with your feeling nervous once in a while. Then you find you rarely ever feel anything *but* nervous, and next thing you know, you're having constant panic attacks—thinking you're going to die because your chest is so tight you can hardly breathe. Or you don't sleep for an entire night. One night turns into a week, and suddenly you haven't slept in eight or 10 days.

When you're faced with these kinds of situations at a young age, you have so little to compare it to. You may wonder if it's normal. You assume it will work itself out. Maybe it's not that big of a deal. But as you fall deeper into the throes of a disorder, it's virtually impossible to remember what "normal" used to feel like. You can't think as clearly as you once did.

Are You a Statistic?

It may seem hard to believe that **one out of five high school students**, and **one out of four college students** suffer from a mental disorder. That's 20% and 25% respectively—pretty significant numbers if you stop to think about it. Imagine a classroom with 100 students. It's possible that 20 to 25 of those students in that class may have some type of mental disorder, and most of them probably don't want you to know, so are feeling pressured to hide it. This only perpetuates the problem.

You lose perspective, making it extremely difficult to compare your newfound moods and behavior to the person you were before the symptoms took hold. It helps to have a period of normalcy to truly realize how bad things have become. However, if you have a mental disorder, "normal" can become too elusive and subjective a term to define.

People may gradually withdraw into silence as their new symptoms take hold. They want to believe that their lives will auto-correct with little or no effort—that the problem will just go away. But it doesn't. Their lives continue to careen out of control, as they try to rationalize their problems with new, creative excuses. And no matter how bad it gets, they refuse to admit they need help. They fear the consequences of what it means to have a disorder, so they continue to say nothing.

MIKE had a hard time recognizing that what was happening to him was related to depression. *It started with me no longer wanting to do the things I enjoyed. Then it became a struggle for me just to leave my room. That's when I started drinking—as my only way to comfortably socialize. My feelings just continued to get worse, but it took a long time for me to even totally recognize it as a serious issue, because on the surface, I basically felt that everyone else was doing what I was doing—we were all drinking, we were all partying. I didn't know I was any different from anyone else. I had just hoped I* would eventually go back to the way I used to be. All of this made it hard for me to identify that I had a real problem.

On the other hand, many people do know they have a problem, but they still refuse to share it with anyone because they fear it will make them a burden.

ANTHONY was a sophomore in college when he finally admitted that he was thinking about taking his own life. *I would fight to make everyone think everything was okay when I was in front of friends or family, but as soon as I was alone, I couldn't stop crying. I started to stay away from my friends after school and only do things with my family when I absolutely had to. Outside of that, I isolated myself and didn't do any of the things I used to like doing.*

My parents got divorced when I was 13. My dad left, and all of a sudden, all of this added pressure was on me. I have four younger brothers and sisters. My mom started placing my dad's old responsibilities on me.

I wanted to make everything okay for our family. I certainly didn't want to burden them with my emotional issues. I figured everyone has problems, right? So why should I talk about mine? If I can't function well for a couple of months, it's not that big of a deal. I just didn't want anyone to have to worry about me.

Thoughts like "*it's not that big of a deal*" are just self-protective justifications to delay your seeking help. You tell yourself that things aren't "that bad," at least not in comparison to what has happened to you so far in life, or especially when you consider what's happening to other people all around the world. You should be able to deal with it on your own. No one will really understand anyway, right? Of course, it's your choice whether to ask for help. But if you don't, and you find that your life isn't improving, you will be increasingly vulnerable to heading down a deep, downward spiral.

"People Will Think I'm Weak"

Embarrassment is a big deal. It's so big that it can even mean the difference between life and death. Talking about your problems can be humiliating, not to mention scary. You may feel afraid of being judged. You may think it will get you into trouble. Or you may believe that "big boys don't cry." Most people feel great pressure to conform to whatever they think is "normal."

ALISON lost her brother to suicide when she was just in her first year of college. *We don't know exactly what the reasons were* *that Brian didn't feel comfortable talking to anyone about having a mental disorder. Since he and I were so similar, though, I've been able to reflect on his situation and get some idea. He was especially brilliant and had been incredibly successful in school. Then, all of a sudden, there was something wrong with his brain—which he saw as his biggest strength. I'm sure he was afraid he might lose his identity as the smart; funny, popular guy everyone knew him to be. I think he probably felt alone and scared, as though he was the only person struggling—maybe he just wasn't sure if anyone would totally understand everything he was feeling.*

The trouble with not talking about your emotions is simply this: it doesn't work. You can only hide your feelings for so long before they come out anyway, in ways that may only end up hurting you. Not talking about your problems is like asking a boiling kettle not to release its steam. It's impossible. Something's got to give.

PAUL witnessed a horrific car accident. A passenger was thrown through the window and decapitated. What's worse is that he later learned the victim was one of his closest friends. *I've always been afraid to talk about how it affected me, seeing my friend killed like that. I go to a really competitive private high school. No one ever talks about emotions like that—it would be seen as a sign of weakness. We all compete at everything, from grades, girls, sports, getting into the best schools, whatever. You never want someone to have something on you—I guess that's mostly why I hide my feelings.*

Not to complain, but my own parents even made me feel sort of like I should ultimately just deal with it and move on with my life. But since my friend died, it's like I'm filled with rage all the time—I just feel like I hate everything. I've been breaking things and punching walls. I drink a lot lately, too—sometimes even to the point of passing out. Overall, I feel like I just don't care about very much anymore.

At first, when you talk about highly charged feelings, it can seem like you've electrified a raw nerve or torn a scab from your skin. It can be really intense. Some of the uncomfortable emotions are bound to linger for a while, which is normal. Problems—and especially mental disorders—cannot magically disappear after a little air time.

Even so, the residual emotions can make you feel week and debilitated, as if you're a total loser. Many people think that talking about something difficult or emotional a time or two should be enough to make the pain go away. That you should then be able to get on with your life and forget about whatever it was that was bothering you. You may berate yourself. "Why can't I just get over it?" It's not that simple, that's why. It's a process that just takes time. Sadly, many people allow the frustration to derail their attempts to work through their issues.

We live in a quick-fix society. But mental disorders and traumatic events do not always have an easy solution.

AMBER was diagnosed with an eating disorder. *Everything is just so competitive all the time. Most people act like if you cry or show emotion or hurt about a lot of things, you're just weak, you need to be tougher, you need to suck it up or something. It's hard to explain, but there was no way for me to just "suck it up" or magically make my eating disorder go away.*

If you have an issue that's negatively affecting you, it's critical to take the time to try to understand what it is, why it's gripping you, and what you can do about it. Talking about your problems can make you feel exposed. It forces you to admit that your issues are real. But in doing so, you'll build a power that is deep and internal—something no one can take away from you.

It *doesn't* mean you're weak. In fact, it actually takes a lot of *strength* and courage to be able to talk about your problems. Much more strength than it takes to drink, do drugs, injure yourself, or just keep everything inside. And by actively participating in your own recovery, you'll discover irrefutable evidence of just how strong you really are.

"I Can't Trust Anyone"

Some of you may read this and think, "but wait, I can trust people—I have over 168 'friends' on my buddy list!" And most people even have that special section devoted to *top* friends or "best friends forever." But when it comes to talking about mental health, suddenly you might find it hard to trust even those people you may think of as your closest friends.

While there may be at least one person in your group of friends who you know you can't trust, there are hopefully others that you can. But remember that real trust doesn't come instantly. Most of you learn this the hard way—only after you've shared your darkest secrets with someone, who later went and told the world. You want to feel closer, so while feeling overly optimistic about a new friend, you invest too much too soon. You end up confiding in someone before they've earned it—before you've learned whether or not they truly have your best interests at heart. When you open up too quickly, you may subconsciously hope that by telling this person everything, your problems will go away, or get better. But you just set yourself up to feel frustrated and disappointed when they persist. And what's more, you make yourself vulnerable to people who may not be good for you.

CYNTHIA had been dealing with depression, attention deficit disorder, and cutting since high school, when her parents split up. *When I first started college, I was excited to meet people and find sup-*

port. Overall, the people I met were very supportive. I made some friends and began to feel a little better—even a little more normal—after the hell of having to survive through high school with all my issues. I practically breezed through the first couple years of college, and moved in with four other women at the start of my junior year.

I started to feel so close to my roommates. We did everything together. One night when I was talking with my roommate Anne, we both talked about a lot of personal things and I ended up sharing a bunch of things with her about my past. I felt like it was something I could safely share with her, so I didn't hold back. I went into every detail about my parents' divorce, my depression, and even the cutting. I cried a lot, as I revealed to her some excruciating details of my story that I had never told anyone else. I did feel vulnerable, but I was also comforted by the fact that someone who cared about me was taking the time to listen. When I woke up the next day though, I started to feel kind of weird about having disclosed so much of my past to Anne, in the sense that I really hadn't known her all that long.

I suddenly felt deathly afraid that Anne would tell someone—if not everyone in our house, so I went to her for reassurance. "I would SO never tell a soul," Anne said, hugging me tightly. I felt bad for ever having doubted her sincerity. She brushed it off, and we made plans to hang out later that week. I went back to my room feeling better—that maybe it was okay to trust her after all.

But the next morning, I woke up again with the same feeling of dread I felt before. I didn't know what to believe—what

Anne had said, or the insecurity I felt from my gut. I went into the kitchen, and Anne was whispering to my other roommates, who were giggling—I heard them saying things like, "No way, what a freak" and "she's such a psycho."

I stood in the doorway, stunned, unable to think of something clever to say—I wanted to say anything I could to erase what I had told Anne, to turn it all into a joke. But the smell of coffee nauseated me. I was so upset in that moment, I started to duck into to the bathroom before any of them saw me, but it was too late.

"Oh, hi, Cynthia," one of my other roommates said, her voice awkward and patronizing. Anne, who had her back to me, spun around quickly.

"Um, hey, Cyn—want some coffee?" she asked. I barely found the breath to say no, and I left the room. As I turned the corner, their gossiping and giggling resumed. Assuming that they were probably still talking about me, I just wanted to die. But the nightmare didn't end there.

When I returned from class that day, someone had left me an anonymous note on my corkboard saying, "Don't worry, we're here for you. You're not alone!" I was devastated. I felt my roommates were mocking me. And later that day I confirmed that they were. Our house erupted into a virulent strain of gossip about me, and everything I had been through. I felt my roommates were constantly talking behind my back about it. After that, I had to wonder if I would ever be able to really trust anyone again.

Did You Know?

You may be surprised to learn that a recent study showed 25% of people in our country feel they have NO ONE who they can confide in. 75% of respondents said they feel that they can confide in just ONE specific person. The same study also showed that only 50% of people in marriages felt they could confide in their partner. (As it happens, the divorce rate is also about 50%, so lack of communication and trust may have something to do with it. What do *you* think?)

Cynthia made a common mistake, one that can happen to anyone, at any age. She had the courage to open up about a painful problem, but she chose the wrong person to confide in, shared too many details too quickly, and then she couldn't go back. She couldn't erase what she'd said. But this doesn't mean that it's impossible for her—or *you*—to trust people in the future.

Trust can take a while to develop, especially during the more difficult periods in your life. You need to take the time to see who is really worthy of your trust, because not everyone is. If you need to find someone to talk to while you're still working on developing new friendships and finding out if you can rely comfortably on the friends you have, there are several resources available, whether you're in high school or college (counselors, clergy members, mental health professionals, hotline services, etc.). These people are professionals. Trustworthiness and maintaining confidentiality is part of their job.

Building trust can be a real challenge at times.

JASON is a high school student in Illinois. *I have a lot of feelings that I'd probably never share because I don't usually feel like I can trust people with things like that. Everyone always treats me like the guy who can solve any type of problem. They only see me as the "tough" football player. It's true that I am the biggest guy in my school by far, no one messes with me, and anyone who has even tried I have thumped pretty badly. But the thing is, people also assume I never have any big problems, when some days I actually feel like I'm going to break down. Most of the time it's like my "exterior life" is the opposite of what I'm really going through inside. Honestly, it's a bummer when you don't have anyone you can really talk to about stuff, you know? But it just seems like no one really wants to believe the idea that I could possibly be going through anything serious.*

The fear of not being able to trust anyone with your true feelings can be very real. But it is possible to find a middle ground—between trusting too quickly (or trusting the wrong people), and just choosing not to trust anyone at all.

If you want to build mutual trust with someone, you need to give it time. You have to open up gradually, so both you and your friend can process what you're revealing. Don't divulge everything about yourself all at once. And no matter how much you may like them or want to be their friend, *don't* confide in someone who is already widely known to be a gos-

BehindHappyFaces.com

sip. If someone routinely gossips about other people, what makes you think they won't also gossip about *you*?

CHRIS was diagnosed with obsessive-compulsive disorder, and finally found a friend he felt comfortable talking to about it. *It's hard to trust other people, especially when you don't totally understand what is happening to you. I wasn't sure of what to say to people about my obsessive-compulsive disorder, so I only talked to one of my close friends about it, gradually confiding in him more as time went on and we felt more sure of each other. I still have a lot of stuff I'm going through trying to manage my disorder, but my friend is there to help me, and over the years I have learned I can absolutely trust him.*

Having someone to talk to—someone you can trust—is crucial. But at the same time, don't expect your friend to be your therapist. Friends can listen and friends can support you, but they cannot single-handedly take your pain away or solve your problems for you.

"I Can't Find the Words"

Have you ever been in a situation where you just don't know what to say? A friend's parent dies. Your parents get divorced. Maybe the words are in your head, but you just don't know where to begin. You think hard, you take your time, you rack your brain. You do everything you can, but no matter how hard you try, you just can't seem to find the right words. We rely on words for so much of our communication, but very often when it comes to life's most challenging moments, we're suddenly mutes.

ROSS *I never did learn how to express my feelings very well. So when I had my first episode with bipolar disorder, I really had no idea how to put my thoughts and feelings about it into words. I was 16, living in a rural small town in Pennsylvania, where no one talked about this stuff. We just didn't have words for these kinds of things. We had alcohol and violence, sure, but we didn't really have words.*

SARAH was raped when she was just 16 years old. *A while after it happened, I was going through a lot and feeling completely out of control of my emotions, but when people asked me how I felt, I didn't know how to describe it. Everyone kept nagging and asking me what was wrong, but it was like I had no ability to tell them, exactly. Not having the words to express myself would make me feel stupid, so then I would shut down even more.*

When you don't know how to express yourself or describe what's happening to you, it doesn't take much to feel embarrassed and want to shut down. But when you keep suppressing powerful emotions, you're *at risk* for acting out. The feelings have to go somewhere—so if you don't talk them out, you'll probably end up acting them out. And we're not talking about an interpretive dance here. Unexpressed emotions have a way of coming out in all kinds of directions. This can often be the cause of excessive drinking, drugging, cutting, and more.

Ross once spoke to a group of students at a Georgia continuation school, where he met Tyrone, a 19-year-old, massive chunk of a guy. Standing 6'5," he looked like someone you wouldn't want to mess with. After Ross concluded his presentation, Tyrone waited for everyone to leave the room. He then approached Ross with an aggressive lunge—and proceeded to scoop him up in a big bear hug. Ross didn't know what to think or how to react. He was actually a little alarmed, not knowing what was going to happen. Really, he just wanted his feet back on the ground. This was a tough school, where gang fights erupt all the time and there's very little security. Ross's ribs smarted from the pressure of Tyrone's powerful embrace. But before Ross could do or say anything, Tyrone suddenly started shaking—and weeping. He put Ross down, and held up his huge fists, the size of cantaloupes.

TYRONE is a 19-year-old gang member. *These hands have punched, stabbed, and beaten more people than I can probably remember. Ever since I was* *little, my dad has been in a gang. When I was only three, he took me on gang fights and beat people with baseball bats in front of me. He and my brothers would constantly beat the crap out of me and say that I would never be tough enough. My dad's in a gang. I grew up in a gang. I'm still in a gang, and I probably always will be.*

I have so many things running through my head all the time, but I usually don't have the words to express them. I have scars—not words. My girlfriend was the one person who could manage to keep me calm. She would try to help me talk through a lot of the stuff on my mind, but she just broke up with me two days ago. I'm pretty messed up about it, and I'm afraid I'm going to go back to violence, beating people or whatever, because I honestly don't know another way to deal with this. Who am I supposed to talk to, and how do I even find the words, anyway?

Tyrone lives in an extreme world that may feel far removed from your own, but the difficulties he has when it comes to sorting through and expressing his feelings are no different from the difficulties so many other people have when they're growing up. Emotions were never discussed in his home, so how could he have known how to describe what was happening to him?

But even if you can't always find the words, you're not trapped with your emotions. If it seems impossible for you to put your thoughts and feelings into words, then you can try other ways of expressing yourself. Maybe it is easier for you to paint, write poetry, freestyle rap, dance. Or maybe it's possible for you to connect to certain lyrics in some of the music that you like. Some people find it helpful to log onto mental health websites where they can interact or read other people's posts about certain issues, as sometimes they find they can relate to what others are going through. Other people might like to read books. The best thing is to find something comfortable that you may even enjoy doing. If you are totally lost or unsure about who you can talk to, remember that you can always go and speak to a counselor. Professionals know the right questions to ask and how to guide you. You may feel weird or scared at first, but truly, nothing is more empowering than finally finding your words—finally discovering how to express your emotions.

When You Can't Stop Hurting Yourself

One of the more dramatic ways to act out unexpressed emotions is through *self-injury*. Self-injury includes almost anything you can do to cause yourself pain: cutting, scratching, picking scabs, burning, punching yourself or objects, infecting yourself, inserting objects in your body openings, bruising or breaking bones, even pulling out your hair, as well as other forms of bodily harm. It's a lot more complicated than just seeking solace in a packet of razor blades, which is how cutting has been depicted in the media. A large majority of cutters also have absolutely no intention of killing themselves. They actually cut to *relieve* the pain, which is difficult for most people to understand.

Self-injury is very complex. There is a tendency to explain it as a "way to remove stress," but more often it is a coping mechanism. Many people who hurt themselves were sexually abused—the more intense the sexual abuse, the harsher the "self-abuse." But it's important to remember that this isn't the case for everyone, and that just because someone cuts, it doesn't necessarily mean he or she has been sexually abused.

Many young people, particularly young women, cut because they want to control their pain. Cutting is an outlet, an unhealthy way to express stress, pain, fear, or anxiety. In his book *Cutting: Understanding and Overcoming Self-Mutilation* (W.W. Norton & Co., 1998), author Dr. Steven Levenkron talks about how young people create an emotional buildup in their minds. The pain becomes intense, and because they have no way of talking about it, they cut themselves. You could say that cutters cry from their arms instead of their eyes. The act of cutting hurts, but afterwards, the physical release (which is really an endorphin rush, a release of pain-easing chemicals into the brain) relieves the emotional pain. And sometimes cutters actually become addicted to these endorphins, which makes cutting extremely difficult for them to stop.

Whether you or someone you know may be cutting, or perhaps just keeping your emotions locked inside because you can't find the words to express them, it is important to know that the words *are* out there. Sometimes it takes a while for us to find them, and many times it even takes the help of a mental health professional to bring them out into the open. Whenever someone first tries to speak about their emotions it can be scary, and may feel easier to just shut down. But just as you need to take the time to learn to trust people, you also need to give yourself time to understand your feelings and how best to express them.

"I Hate Myself"

JULIE was just nine years old when her parents got divorced. She's now a sophomore in college. *My parents played favorites and tried to get us to turn against one another. I still feel so guilty about my parents' divorce. I feel like it was totally my fault. And I don't like admitting this, but I truly hate myself for it.*

Divorce was enough to trigger Julie's self-loathing, and stories like this are not uncommon. So many people out there feel this way. Painful life events—like the diagnosis of a mental disorder, a divorce, death, breakup, rejection, isolation, or even seemingly smaller disappointments can derail you—if not totally incapacitate you. The change can be very disruptive, causing many different reactions. It's like suddenly you don't know where you end and the problem begins. You blame yourself. You become hostile, angry, and bitter. You isolate yourself, directing inward all the anger that you feel. You feel as though everything is your fault. You feel worthless, and anything that happens from that point forward may serve to deepen the intensity of your self-hate. Eventually, you may feel like giving up. Because when you hate yourself, it's hard to see a reason to keep trying. And when that happens, you're less likely to seek help.

What Can I Do If I Hate Myself?

Self-hatred is a common by-product of mental disorders, mental health issues and even just life itself. Your *best* defense is to build up your self-esteem. What do you like best about yourself?

• Make a list of 10 best qualities. If not 10, then how about *one*?

• Find out what your friends and family value about you. If you don't know, then how about just asking them?

• If you can only think of one positive thing that you like about yourself, don't stress. That's a good start! Over time, and with increased self-awareness, that one quality will grow and evolve into several more, and you will begin to feel better about yourself. Focusing on your self-worth is a major building block of recovery.

If You're Scared to Seek Help

In this chapter we've outlined the most common reasons why many young people don't talk about their problems. Obviously these aren't the only reasons, but chances are, you know them well. You may live them every day—hiding behind a happy face, pretending to be fine when you're hurting inside, or maybe you're just too shut down emotionally to feel much of anything. The resistance you feel about discussing your inner turmoil is universal. It's actually even normal. Opening up can be uncomfortable, if not embarrassing. It can totally derail your concept of who you are and where you think your life is heading. For some of us, it's pretty scary stuff.

But here's the good news – while you've been turning inside out at the mere thought of ever talking about your "stuff," the medical community has developed safe and effective treatment programs. By the time you're ready to deal with yourself, they're ready for *you*. There are so many resources available today to help someone who wants the support, it's actually almost mind-boggling. But the thing is, you have to want it. There's no "dialing in" your recovery.

If you truly want to get better, you'll have to deal with the reasons that have been keeping you from addressing your issues. We all have our reasons—parents, family, friends, experiences—or maybe it's just the stigma of having a problem. Any one of these reasons is enough to keep us isolated. But once you identify your reasons for *not* wanting to seek help, you have a better chance of working through it.

Half the battle is understanding yourself.

If Someone You Know Is Scared to Seek Help

If you think you know someone who needs help, but is avoiding the issue, then it may be helpful to uncover his or her reasons. But you must be patient. Mental disorders can cloud a person's ability to analyze the reasons behind their resistance to seeking help. Even so, it's an important conversation to have. If you don't know what to say to them or how you can help, consider talking to a school counselor, social worker, psychologist or any mental health professional about what your friend or family member is going through. They can try to help you find the right approach.

It may be challenging to get someone to open up emotionally. You may encounter intense resistance. It could get ugly. Or uncomfortable. Or the person could be surprisingly receptive, maybe even relieved, wondering why it took you so long to muster the courage to open your mouth. You just never know, so you have to plan accordingly. And also remember that many times people are only asked to talk about their emotions *after* they have been diagnosed with a disorder or experienced a life-changing event. If the person never talked about his or her emotions *before* something serious happened, then it could be excessively uncomfortable to discuss emotions *afterward*. But these feelings can be strong. And when emotions bottle up inside with nowhere to go, people sometimes feel as if their bodies have been hijacked. (And they have no idea who's driving.)

If you run into difficulty, don't feel as though you need to pressure them. It might go a long way just to simply assure them that you care about them, and that you are willing to listen whenever they might need to talk to someone.

Help Is Out There

There is often a rush to get someone with a mental disorder the proper treatment, medication, or diagnosis. This is important, but you may not be as comfortable with these things if you don't identify the reasons why you have been avoiding seeking help. Understanding why it was so hard to ask for that help when you needed it will actually make it easier to *get* help, and easier for others to help you.

Wouldn't it be easy to talk about your feelings if your shinbone snapped in two and suddenly popped through your skin? Ouch. You'd have quite a lot to say about it—and pretty loudly, too. Well, the brain is no different. Legs can break. Brains can run off track. Bodies can malfunction. If you break your shinbone, you may limp around for a bit, but chances are that if you adhere to your doctor's plan and refrain from performing high jumps for a while, you will heal.

Pain is pain. It's universal. It's life. It happens every day, and there's not much you can do to avoid it. If anything, try to embrace it. Talk about it. And find somebody to help you with it, exactly the way you'd find a doctor to set your broken leg. The more you do this, the stronger you'll be. For yourself, or maybe for that friend—the one who's always pretending to be happy (when you know there's more going on inside). In the upcoming chapters, we'll get into more specifics on exactly how to get help, and how to best utilize it when you do.

CHAPTER 3

NO ONE IS ALONE:
Gender, Race, Class & Sexuality

"We are so accustomed to disguise ourselves to others, that in the end we become disguised to ourselves."
—*François de la Rochefoucauld,*
French author & moralist (1613–1680)

ROSS *On January 5ᵗʰ of my senior year I was hospitalized for wanting to take my own life. The scary thing is that nothing unusual happened on THAT particular day. I woke up and went to school. After school I had a basketball game. After we won the game, I went to a restaurant with my friends, just like we always did. And on the way home from the restaurant—I decided I no longer wanted to live.*

What is important to note about that is that most people who take (or attempt to take) their own lives DON'T WANT TO DIE. They just can't handle living the way they are living anymore, and taking their own life is a sure way out of it. In my case, I didn't really want to die, but I also couldn't handle thinking about death and suicide constantly, either. I honestly believed that my parents, friends, and everyone close to me would be better off if I were gone. I thought that I was somehow relieving them of my life. That wasn't the reality of course, but it's how I felt at that time.

Luckily, my parents managed to get me to the hospital before anything too major happened. But that night, I flipped out and the nurses had to give me a tranquilizer. I woke up about 24 hours later, to find I had no drawstrings in my sweatshirts, no shoelaces in my shoes, and no sheets on my bed. There was also someone watching me at all times. A couple of days after that, we had group therapy. Everyone was supposed to talk about why they were there. The stories before mine were filled things like sexual abuse, physical abuse, suicides in the family.

When it was my turn to speak I didn't know WHAT to say. I really didn't know exactly why I had thought I wanted to die. So they asked me to tell them about myself. I said, "Hi, my name is Ross. I was the president of my junior class. I played varsity basketball for two years. I was a member of Peer Helper and S.A.D.D. I volunteered five years with the Special Olympics, helped the physically challenged during my study halls, attended the National Young Leaders Conference, I have a 3.6 GPA..." and finally, I stopped. Just then, I felt really stupid! The life I was describing was my external life. The life everyone else saw, but NOT the life that I was living. If I wanted to talk about the life I was living, I should have said, "Hi, my name is Ross, and I hate myself. I don't think anyone should care about me. Most of the people important to me have already left anyway..."

After I got out of the hospital, I went back to high school. But everything had changed. BEFORE I went into that hospital, I was a cool guy. I was someone people partied with, the guy everyone liked. But after I got out of the hospital, I was suddenly a "loony," "wacko," "psycho...the "crazy" kid. I was now the guy people made fun of, and ultimately I was the guy who lost friends.

Two months after my release from the hospital, a psychologist visited my classroom, and he spoke about some of the types of patients he was treating. As he told extreme stories of people with mental disorders, almost everyone in the class began to laugh. But I wasn't laughing. I was angry. I pulled my teacher aside and we went into the hallway. I told him that I had bipolar disorder, and didn't think this was funny. He asked me what I wanted to do about my classmates' laughter, and I asked him if he would let ME speak.

So two weeks later, he put me in front of the class and I gave my first speech. In some ways, it was easily—one of THE worst experiences of my life! My knees were shaking. I was sweating in areas I didn't know could sweat. I stood gripping the podium, just hoping to make it through. But interestingly, when I finished my speech, nobody laughed. More importantly, some people even came up to me afterward and started sharing similar stories within their own families ("my brother..." "my sister..." "my mother..." "my friend..."). They told me stories of loved ones who committed suicide or other family members being diagnosed with mental illnesses. Some asked me if I knew where they could go for help, because they were experiencing some of the same symptoms. So I learned at a young age that speaking about these issues wasn't only good for me, but helpful for so many others as well.

Common Negative Stereotypes About Mental Illness

The friends who deserted Ross after he got out of the hospital, and the students in his class who were laughing—these people were only thinking about the extreme stereotypes of mental illness, that people with mental disorders must be "crazy" or dangerous. But they stopped laughing when they heard the truth from one of their own peers who was living with it. After hearing Ross' truth, they found it easier to acknowledge some truths about mental health in their own lives. Here are some other common and unfortunate stereotypes about mental health.

- *All women are highly emotional and have an easy time talking about their feelings.*

- *Men aren't capable of talking about emotion.*

- *It's not acceptable to talk openly about mental health issues or mental disorders.*

- *People with money don't have as many problems as other people.*

- *Poor people can't seek help.*

- *Being gay or lesbian is a mental disorder.*

You may agree with some of the above statements, and you may also think there isn't anything wrong with that. But let's take a closer look at these stereotypes and decide how true they really are.

Did You Know?

Over 57 million American adults are affected by one or more mental disorders each year.

What You Don't Know About Women

It's a common misconception that all women can talk easily and comfortably about their feelings. The media floods us with images of women routinely chatting on about the most intimate things in their personal lives, as if there's nothing to it. So when it comes to mental health issues, you'd think that if this were the case, women must have it easier, right? Wrong. Deep emotions can be just as difficult for women to share as it is for many men. Don't assume that women never feel that they have to keep their innermost feelings to themselves. Many of them do.

While women may be widely encouraged to talk about their emotions, sometimes when they *can't* express them for whatever reason, they feel even worse about their situation,

The Truth About Men and Women and Mental Disorders

- Women are more likely to experience depression than males.

- Women are more likely to attempt suicide, but males are more likely to die from it.

- Women are more likely to develop an eating disorder than young men.

- As many as 10 million women currently suffer from anorexia and bulimia. Approximately 25 million more suffer from binge eating disorder. Eating disorders are among the deadliest and most difficult mental disorders to treat.

- Women are two times as likely to experience generalized anxiety disorder.

- Women are more likely than men to seek help for their problems.

Why are women more at risk? There are several reasons. For one, women are more often the victims of sexual abuse. Females also deal with radical shifts in hormones. Some women are influenced by society's superficial and unrealistic expectations—thinking they have to be impossibly beautiful like the women they see on magazines or TV—and then berating themselves when they fall short.

And that's just the physical component. Emotionally, women feel just as much pressure to be perfect—to "please." They're expected to have careers and raise children, to be virginal and sexy... it's no wonder so many young women are left feeling conflicted, inadequate, or overwhelmed. Many are led to believe that they should be seen and not heard, that pleasing others is more important than asserting themselves, and that so long as they're always "perfect," they'll never be alone. These self-limiting beliefs in combination with the stigma already surrounding mental disorders can have a powerfully negative effect—which is why so many women are hesitant to admit their problems.

as if they've failed in some way. Since it's just assumed to be so easy for women to share emotion, then if a woman has difficulty, it just further fuels her perception that something must be wrong with her. In some cases, however, a woman can fall victim to the opposite stereotype—one that says it's wrong for her to even *have* real needs or emotions at all.

MARTHA was diagnosed with depression. **Her mother had schizophrenia.** *As women, we are taught to value sacrifice, especially for our families. My father made it very clear to me when I was eight or nine years old that he needed to depend on me to help him out with my mom while she was sick. I wasn't supposed to act like a kid anymore—I had to be the good, responsible daughter. I think I was even given some examples from the Bible to inspire me to take on this role (my family was very religious at the time).*

Even as a kid, I was never allowed to cry. If I did, it made my father very uncomfortable and he would make fun of me, calling me a "baby." Or he would patronize me by saying things like, "You look much prettier when you don't cry." All of which was very confusing to me. My looks were never really discussed at that age unless I was crying, which was such a weird context. I really didn't know how to take that. I remember how just the confusion alone would sometimes be enough to get me to stop crying.

I didn't finally seek help until I was in college. My friends begged me to see a doctor about my emotional health. If it hadn't been for them, I would probably still be suppressing my feelings. I was ultimately diagnosed with depression, but I refused to accept the label for fear of ending up like my mother. After a year, school ended and I went back into denial. I began numbing out with alcohol, weed and occasionally even having sex with men I didn't care about.

I didn't start therapy again until I had another massive bout with depression a couple of years later. I happened upon a women's group in Greenwich Village that was run by a psychotherapist. A few months later, I started seeing the psychotherapist for private sessions and taking prescribed medication. I've had a few relapses since that time, but have always been conscious of what was going on and have managed to take steps to heal myself or seek out support and treatment when I've needed it.

All of these things—feeling like you have to be perfect, or that it's not okay to have or express your own needs—can make it particularly hard for women and girls to talk about emotions. And even if you *do* open up about how you truly feel, you aren't always taken seriously as a female. You're a "drama queen." You're "too emotional." It must be "that time of the month..." These are just a few of the responses women can hear when sharing their true feelings. It's almost as if— just because you're a woman—your emotions are less valid. But talking about emotion should never be taken lightly. It's much healthier to feel, cry, release and express what is happening, than it is to hold it all in.

Big Boys *Do* Cry (and Can "Hug It Out")

Imagine a world where men and boys actually talk, cry, embrace, resolve conflicts, and express more emotion than anyone has ever thought imaginable. This isn't a dream. What we've just described is what occurs at major sporting events across the country every day.

There is a widespread belief that men never talk about emotion, and some people believe they don't even *feel* emotion. But think about it. If you've ever been to a big game, you know that's not true. Every person—male *or* female—has feelings. There is a huge difference between men not having emotion, and men not feeling comfortable *expressing* emotions. In the stereotypical man's world, it's generally okay to express emotion for your favorite team, at a wedding (so long as it's your own and not someone else's), or maybe a funeral—but that's about it. It can be exceptionally difficult to get young men to address personal emotions in situations in which they are not comfortable.

Men are typically reluctant to reveal their innermost feelings. But when dealing with symptoms of a mental disorder, they can feel even more uncomfortable.

ROSS   *I didn't know how to talk about how I felt. My parents never really talked about emotions. My mom grew up in a home where she was expected to get through things on her own. My dad grew up in a similar environment, so I didn't get much help there either. My friends were noticing something was going on with me, but I felt I couldn't tell them anything. Many times they just thought it was kind of funny if I flipped out or did something stupid. I discovered it was easier for me to act out in outlandish ways rather than sit down and talk about what was really happening. Unfortunately, for me, that led to way too much binge drinking. In my area, it was always cool to see who could drink the most and who could be the most self-destructive.*

I also found that drinking seemed to be a much more acceptable way for me to deal with what was happening to me, than actually talking about it. If I did try to tell people what was happening, I would often get a lot of weird looks or condescending comments. However, if I drank too much and became emotional or cried, then of course it was "just the alcohol." I can't say that all of this was coming from my friends or family. A lot of it was just in my own head, and while members of my family would say things like "Suck it up" or "Be a man," those kinds of comments would only reinforce my existing beliefs.

Even though it can be difficult for men to talk about their mental health issues, they definitely have them. We all do. And mental health does differ between men and women. Research suggests that men are more likely than women to abuse alcohol or to act out in other self-destructive ways in order to ease their pain. They are also more likely to suffer from antisocial behavior, which can lead to fighting, becoming withdrawn, or not knowing how to go about developing friendships or relationships. Some experts believe that more men are starting to experience eating disorders and problems with body image. This may be fueled by the increasing use of steroids in male high school and college students as they strive to appear stronger, fitter, and tougher. A lot of high schools and colleges report an increase in young men cutting themselves. Some mental health professionals also believe that men experience the same number of mental disorders as women, but have a much lower rate of seeking help.

Physical Pain = Emotional Pain

Coping mechanisms that people develop at a young age can affect them for the rest of their lives. In a recent study, researchers at the UCLA School of Psychology measured what areas of the brain are affected when someone experiences excessive physical pain like losing an arm or having an eye gouged. They discovered that the same areas of the brain that are affected during physical pain are also affected when someone faces a social rejection. Which just goes to show, emotional pain is every bit as real to us as physical pain.

But men don't behave this way just because they're male. They do it because to some extent, it's how they've been taught. When boys can grow up seeing their male role models *talking* about how they feel—instead of hiding from emotions or problems—then they may be more likely to follow suit.

ADAM grew up in an open home environment. *My dad is a psychologist, so when I was growing up, he was always concerned with how I felt and what was going on with me. From the earliest time, I can remember he would talk to me about the more difficult things that none of my other friends' parents would discuss, stuff like sex, drinking and drugs. He never condoned any of it, but he was more interested in why my friends and I may be doing it. Being able to talk about stuff helped me identify a lot of things about myself. This isn't to say that I didn't ever drink or do any of those things, but I was generally more in touch with my feelings than most of my friends were. Some people may have thought I was weird because of that, but I felt a lot more stable than most of the people I knew.*

Adam was raised in a world where it was okay to express his feelings, which isn't the norm. Most men are taught – either by society or their own family and friends – that any display of emotion is a sign of weakness. If you succumb, it means you're soft. You're a "pussy." Some guys will go so far as to call other guys "gay" if and when feelings are revealed. (As if straight guys never feel anything!)

It's sad what the fear of emotion can do to guys. Ross was once asked to speak at a college that had four fraternity-related suicides in just one semester. None of the fraternities' members came to the presentation, even though attendance was required. Later, when some of the guys were asked why they didn't show up, they said they didn't want to sit around talking about what happened—that talking about emotions and stuff is "weak." And this was after having lost four people to suicide in four short months! It's not only in fraternities where you'll find the stereotype that emotion equals weakness. But the truth is, it takes a lot more strength to talk about and face negative situations than it does to turn to alcohol, violence, drugs, or shutting your emotions down altogether.

But there are some men out there who have found healthy ways to express their emotions. Sometimes they are just more comfortable because of the way they were raised. Other times, they are forced to learn because it's the only way they are able to deal with a mental disorder or traumatic life experience. But when this doesn't happen, emotion comes out all too often in self-destructive ways that men may feel are more acceptable somehow—drinking, drugs, violence.

If you have a male friend or relative who is having trouble expressing his feelings, what can you do to help him feel more comfortable? There really isn't a 10-step plan on how to make every guy feel at ease, but it's no surprise that a lot of young men may feel more comfortable talking with their female friends or girlfriends. Some consider it more acceptable to open up to a woman than to another man. Look in chapters four, five, and six for specific suggestions on how you can help the people in your life feel more comfortable talking about their problems.

RICK is 19 years old, and when he was in high school he was diagnosed

with bipolar disorder and anger control problems. *It took me a long time to open up about how I was feeling. My parents always tried to get me to talk. My girlfriend was there for me too, but it still felt weird and uncomfortable to open up about stuff. Over time, I learned to open up very slowly. Eventually I was able to get to the point where I can now talk about a lot of what I'm going through, rather than just doing something impulsive or negative—like punching my fist into a wall just to release my frustration.*

Does Race Matter?

One of the most common things we ran into when we would tell people we were writing a book about mental health issues is people who said they typically don't talk about such things at all—that it wasn't really considered acceptable in their community or culture. African-Americans, Latinos, Asians, Arabs, Native Americans, Caucasians—people of nearly every race and ethnicity will often say this. So many people are convinced that nobody in their particular community talks about mental issues. But the truth is, problems with mental health affect all of us in every community—and nearly *everyone* has a hard time talking about them.

So does race have an impact with regard to mental health? In some senses, no. Mental health is an issue for everybody, everywhere. But in some ways, race *does* come into play. A lack of research, advocacy, and minority mental health professionals can make it harder for some minorities to find the help they need. Typically, when people seek help, they prefer to work with someone from a similar race, gender, or class. So minorities may feel that they are at somewhat of a disadvantage, since there are not as many of them currently represented in the mental health field. This could be a significant reason why some minorities don't seek mental health care.

Did You Know?

A national survey revealed that out of the 596 licensed psychologists with active clinical practices who are members of the American Psychological Association, only 1% of the randomly selected sample identified themselves to be Latino. African Americans comprise less than 4% of mental health care providers nationally. In the late 1990s, approximately 70 Asian-American providers were available for every 100,000 Asian Americans in the U.S.

Advocacy organizations, personal stories, and books written by and for minorities are growing, especially in the past decade as more people become aware of the urgency of mental health issues. While this growth is definitely a positive step forward, there is still a major lack of resources and awareness that is hard to miss. In 2004, Ross went to hear Tupac Shakur's mother, Afeni Shakur, speak at the signing of her new book. Someone in the audience asked Afeni if she thought that reviving the Black Panthers would be a good idea. (Afeni was a former member.) She calmly smiled and responded by saying that she felt the most important thing anyone could do is to start going into the high schools and middle schools in minority communities and talking about mental health issues. She said that when she was growing up, it was almost unimaginable for someone to commit suicide, but yet six of Tupac's friends have killed themselves, and she hears more stories like this every day.

Talking about suicide, depression, bipolar disorder, or simply about mental health is hard for anybody—regardless of where you were born, where your parents were born, what language you speak, or what faith you practice. But these things are a fact of life, so being able to talk to someone about how you feel is always the first step toward getting help. And keep in mind that there are a great number of mental health professionals out there ready and willing to help you, so if you know you need to speak to someone, try not to let concerns about race or ethnicity stand in your way. Everyone has equal rights—when it comes to taking charge of our mental health.

Don't Be Fooled By The Rocks That They Got

J-Lo made this phrase famous in her song, "Jenny From The Block." Who can disagree with her? Just because someone has money doesn't mean that person is immune to pain or personal problems. Biggie Smalls was on to something when he said, "Mo' Money, Mo' Problems." Money will never protect you from pain or problems. Life comes with issues for every-body—rich or poor.

Our country is uber-materialistic. Watch MTV for a few minutes and you're flooded with images of Hummers with spinning rims, singers in fur coats and platinum chains, hot bodies dripping in diamonds, prancing through mansions with hundreds of rooms. We idolize wealth. It's the epitome of the American Dream. Unfortunately, along with this comes the assumption that if you have a lot of money, you will have fewer problems or possibly not have to deal with emotional issues at all. Nothing could be further from the truth.

Young people in elite schools are under a lot of pressure to be at the top of their class, get into the best colleges, and land the most distinguished jobs. These pressures can lead to stress, lack of sleep, and overall fear of failure, placing them at a huge risk for mental health issues. Yes, young people from families with money can more easily afford therapy, medication, treatment and psychological help. But they still have to deal with the stigma that comes with admitting they have a problem. Parents may feel that seeking help for a mental disorder could hurt their child's chances of getting into a top college or landing a good job. Students may fear what it will do to their social lives. Having money doesn't mean it's easy to get help.

And now there's a scarier trend, on the opposite end of the spectrum. In some areas of the country, it has almost become a status symbol to have mental health problems. Who would have guessed that seeing two therapists and taking medication would be something that was considered "cool?" But it's happening for some people. The trouble with that is, why would someone want to give up a status symbol by actually getting well? It's alarming when it's cooler to cut yourself, have depression, and be taking a slew of medications than it is to *deal with your issues, take care of yourself, and find your way back to health.*

Did You Know?

Wealthy suburban adolescents have been shown to be at greater risk for depression and drug use than middle-class and lower-class samples of young people. One study showed that more adolescents from privileged families reported using drugs as a means to "escape from problems" or to "relax." In general, they were more likely to use drugs as a way to cope with distress. Urban adolescents typically reported using drugs to "have fun," or because of peer pressure.

Does Being Poor Mean There's No Hope for Me?

On the opposite end of having all of the money in the world, living in poverty *sucks*. No matter how you slice it, when you're struggling to find enough money to buy groceries, it's hard to focus on mental problems, even if you have them and can no longer function normally.

Unfortunately, the high cost of mental health care presents a huge barrier for many people. Middle and lower class families feel this the most, even when both parents work. It can be difficult to afford a good insurance policy – many of which don't even cover all mental health-related costs.

CHERYL, a Chinese American, is recovering from an eating disorder. *My mother has suffered from paranoid schizophrenia with obsessive compulsive tendencies for 30 years. I have binge eating disorder. However, living in a lower-middle class family with only my father working and no insurance made it almost impossible for either of us to seek proper help. It was only in the past couple of years, with the expansion of the mental health system, that we've been fortunate enough to find treatment.*

It was an individual responsibility of mine to research all of my options for finding psychological help for the uninsured, and to be honest, it was a daunting task. I continued to search endlessly on the Internet and by making phone calls. But it was well worth the effort. It took me weeks to find someone who could help us, but I did. I was able to find a psychiatrist for my mother who was fluent in Chinese, as well as a clinic that specified in eating disorders. They also had a sliding scale for the uninsured.

Fortunately, Cheryl managed to find help for herself and her mother, but her story is hardly typical. When it comes to mental health care, it can be hard to find insurance policies with thorough mental health coverage. Oftentimes you'll find that the right medication isn't covered, that you're limited to a certain list of therapists, none of whom may even live in your area. Dealing with the frustration is almost enough to *cause* a mental disorder! Meanwhile, your environment and financial difficulties, in combination with other factors, can be stressful enough to trigger related problems if you're already in need of help. For example, if you're dealing with substance abuse and can't find assistance, you could start to also experience depression.

Cheryl had to overcome a lot of challenges to ultimately find help. Luckily, she was willing to educate herself on these issues. She searched diligently to find what she and her family could do to find treatment. Since she lives in Queens, New York, there were more options available to Cheryl than there might have been if she had lived in a smaller town. Fortunately, however, there are more community resources springing up all over the country. The treatment may not be the best available, but help is coming—and it's certainly better than having to struggle entirely on your own. And if you're in college, you should have a counseling center with anywhere from two to eight free visits, and insurance offered by the school. Getting help shouldn't have to be nearly the challenge for you that it was for Cheryl.

When you are living in a lower class community, sometimes it pays to be creative when dealing with mental health issues. A shining example of how poor communities can sometimes heal is shown in the documentary film, *Rize*. In the movie, filmmaker David LaChappelle documents a dance phenomenon from South Central Los Angeles called "krumping." While it has become infamous in music videos, most people are unaware of its origin. The form of dance became an escape for young people growing up in the extremely poor areas of Watts and other Los Angeles neighborhoods. At the Los Angeles Film Festival screening, one of the dancers eloquently described what krumping meant to him. He told the audience that young people in his neighborhood have to regularly deal with shootings, gangs, absent parents, drugs, alcohol, and a lot of other painful issues. He said it's easy to slip up and not see a way out, because there are so few positive examples available to them. He then explained that for him, krumping *is* a way out. It's a way to express himself and let go of all the BS he has to deal with on a daily basis. In his neighborhood, the only social choice is to either join a gang or dance, and he chooses to dance.

Scenes from the movie show groups of young people having something like a cathartic, emotional breakdown as they dance for the first time, and the positive effect from the community appears to be overwhelming. Now, this is not to say that you can just dance your depression or bipolar disorder away, but it does show that no matter what your financial situation is, young people can be resilient and search to find their own positive ways to cope with the difficulties in their lives.

Sexual Orientation

When it comes to sexual identity and mental disorders, Ross hears all different types of comments and questions from people every day. Do gay people have more mental health issues? How does hiding your sexuality affect your mental health? Is being gay a mental disorder? My friend is gay and has depression—what can I say to him?

To get some answers, we turned to the *Trevor Project*. The Trevor Project is a non-profit organization in Los Angeles that was named in honor of a comedy/drama about a 13-year-old boy who, when rejected by friends and peers because of his sexuality, attempts to take his life. The Trevor Project's mission is to promote acceptance of gay and questioning teenagers and to aid in suicide prevention among that group. (Their website and phone number are in the back of this book.)

Brian Goldman, their program and outreach director, spoke with us about the specific problems people in the LGBTQ (Lesbian, Gay, Bisexual, Transgender and Questioning) community face when dealing with mental health issues.

"It is very possible there is a double stigma among individuals in the LGBTQ community who also happen to have a mental disorder," Goldman says. "Up until the 1970s, being gay or lesbian *was* considered a mental disorder. Those struggling with their sexuality and a diagnosed mental disorder might easily feel as though they are being looked down upon or ridiculed because of their sexuality *and* their mental state. The reality is that there continues to be a stigma surrounding these things. Hopefully, society will gradually become more accepting and understanding of the LGBTQ community, as well as all of those out there suffering from mental disorders."

When someone facing a mental disorder also has issues with their sexual orientation, it may be that much tougher for them to ask for help. "This truly depends on the person," Goldman says. "Dealing with sexuality is already anxiety-provoking, and when an individual suffers from a mental disorder, this only manifests their anxiety to a greater degree. So I do think issues with sexuality can affect a person's willingness to seek the help they need."

There can also be a great deal of guilt or feelings of uncertainty if you haven't yet come out about your sexuality to your friends or family. Which is only natural—you are not only hiding how you feel—you are hiding your true self.

Deathly afraid of the reactions you'll receive, you don't even know where to begin with the conversation. You wonder if you'll lose the love or support of your friends—you may even worry that you'll be disowned by your family. Struggling with any aspect of your personal life can be difficult and lead to massive amounts of stress, uncertainty, and pain. But when someone is forced to hide his or her sexual identity, it can also lead to self-hate, which is often expressed through alcohol, drugs, or other negative means. There is no evidence to suggest that people in the LGBTQ community have a higher rate of mental disorders, but obviously anytime anyone—gay or straight—is hiding a life-altering secret, they will be more vulnerable to acting out by exhibiting unhealthy behavior.

The Real Truth: Mental Health is an Equal-Opportunity Issue

There are endless stereotypes that are applied to people of varying gender, race, class or sexuality. Regardless of which group you may belong to, the real truth is that people in *any* group can find help with their mental issues and will respond to treatment. It's time to finally drop the labels and deal with the truth—whatever that means for you.

Whenever you make a sweeping statement that generalizes about a huge group of human beings—*"Men don't cry,"* *"Nobody in my community ever talks about mental illness,"* *"Women are too emotional,"* etc.—you're almost bound to be wrong some (if not most) of the time. But one truth that does actually apply to every human being is this: mental health is a concern for each one of us. It's not always easy, but problems with mental health can be dealt with—no matter your race, gender, religion, culture, sexuality, or anything else. The first step toward preserving *your* mental health is to stop hiding your pain behind a happy face—and finally start talking to someone about your feelings and your pain. That's the truth.

CHAPTER 4

SURVIVING THE STORM:
Dealing With a Mental Disorder

"So cradle your head in your hands
and breathe, Just breathe, oh breathe,
Just breathe"

—Anna Nalick, "Breathe (2 AM)"

ROSS *After I graduated from high school, I chose to attend American University in Washington, D.C. I arrived on campus that August just like every other college freshman. I was excited about starting over, moving on, going to a place where no one knew anything about me or my past. And I had never lived* *next to girls, so I was like, "hey, this is awesome!" Then about two weeks into my freshman year I started thinking that maybe I should change some things—that maybe I should try being more open about what I was dealing with in my life.*

So one day, I'm sitting at a table with four guys who I had only known for two weeks. At one point during the conversation I blurted out, "So…here's the thing. I've been diagnosed with bipolar disorder with anger control problems and psychotic features. I was actually just hospitalized for wanting to take my own life eight months ago." Hmmm. Can you say…AWK-WARD? After a brief pause, one of the guys turned to me and said, "OK…so…do you need a beer, or a shot?" Another looked at me and said, "Dude. What you need is to hook up with someone." It was real "guy talk", you know…we were having a real, deep, emotional conversation about feelings…

Seriously though, a lot of people struggling with mental health issues will often say, "Nobody ever knew what to do for me." And that was also true for me, but what was more important was that I didn't even really know what I needed to do for MYSELF.

Let's be honest. I came to college with issues. Pretty severe ones. But instead of having a PLAN or finding out where I could go or who I could go talk to if I needed help, I just kind of hoped it would all be okay. What I did was essentially the equivalent of showing up at college in a wheelchair, and hoping they would have ramps.

So whenever I didn't know how to deal with things, my coping mechanism was always to turn to alcohol. Three weeks into my freshman year, I had to get my stomach pumped because of alcohol poisoning. Two months in, I had a relapse with bipolar disorder that was so severe I had to go back home. I was experiencing extreme mania, large outbursts of anger—I was even hearing voices, repeatedly telling me to kill myself.

When I came home, I was hospitalized again. This time when I got out of the hospital, I was very low. I didn't think I had a future. I didn't feel I was capable of anything. I used to sleep on my couch for 18 hours a day or sit out in my backyard and stare out at nothing. I felt like the biggest mess-up and failure in the whole world. I felt like bipolar disorder had won out, and that there was nothing more I could do about it.

My parents encouraged me to take two classes at a community college and work at a restaurant. Later, I took a semester off and got a job working at a warehouse. Then I went to Moravian College near my house for three more semesters. Then I took another year off from school. The whole time, I was trying to figure out what was going to work best for me. Eventually, I decided to return to American University, four years after I originally started.

My first semester back, I thought I was doing okay. But while I was doing well in my classes, I was unfortunately still drinking heavily. And by" heavily," I mean a case of beer every night on the weekends, and a six-pack during the week. One night, towards the end of that first semester, I had over 13 shots in an hour—and then I went out! I consumed more alcohol. I passed out that night at 2 a.m. When I woke up the next day my clock said 12:00, but when I looked outside it was dark. It wasn't noon—it was midnight. I had been passed out for 22 HOURS. I'm sorry to say, this wasn't the first time I had done something like this.

But when I woke up that night, I looked in the mirror and I started to cry. I thought to myself, "Okay, ENOUGH. You are either going to continue this pattern and DIE, or you are going to make a change. Period." I chose to change that night, but change isn't easy. It isn't quick—and it isn't fun. It's definitely not what it appears to be in the movies or on daytime talk shows. No sun shining or bluebirds or any of that. Real change takes a lot of work and a lot of time. But if you want it, I'm here to tell you that you can achieve it.

When dealing with mental disorders, you constantly hear about the medication, the treatment, the diagnosis. As if to say that if you just get those things right, you'll be fine. But it's not as simple as that. While these things are vital, they weren't the biggest problems for me. My biggest problem was that I hated myself. I hated myself because of my bipolar disorder, having to leave school, not getting along with my family, and a long list of other reasons. Because I hated myself, it didn't matter so much what the diagnosis or treatment were. I didn't care enough about myself to even want to take my medications or do whatever else people wanted me to do.

I was also in a massive state of denial. For an entire year before I went back to American University, I went around telling everyone I ever knew from high school and in my hometown that I never had bipolar disorder. That it had all been a big mistake and that everyone, including my doctor, had been wrong. A lot of people actually believed me, but after this last *near-death drinking escapade I felt I couldn't deny my disorder or dysfunction any longer.*

So the first thing I needed to deal with was my self-hatred. I needed to learn to like myself again. The way I did this was to try to focus on one thing I liked about myself during those times of immense self-hatred, and then build up from there. My friends also helped me by being there for support and reminding me what they liked about me, but I had to want to see it myself.

After I learned to like myself more, then I found I could deal much more easily with my bipolar disorder. I had to adhere to my treatment, but more importantly, I had to change some things in my personal life. I had to stop binge drinking. (Kind of a no-brainer there.) I had to stop smoking cigarettes. Stop smoking weed. Start exercising. I had to put myself on a schedule where I would go to sleep and wake up at the same time every day. I stopped drinking caffeine. (I haven't had a coffee or soda in six years.) I also had to structure my life so that I could learn more about my warning signs, recognize what was mania or depression and what to do about it, so I could talk to my doctor or whomever, when I needed to.

Determining *YOUR* Best Action Plan

Dealing with a mental disorder is a complex, lifelong process. There are no quick fixes, magic bullets, or easy solutions for getting well. Regardless of what you want to believe, it won't happen overnight. There is no file to download. No subscription. Nor can you talk, trick, dance, or negotiate your way out of a mental disorder. And the way you ultimately choose to deal with it will profoundly affect your future.

This book doesn't have a 10-step plan for you to follow. The following tips are based on the main concerns we've heard from thousands of other young people, the collective advice of many in the mental health community, and Ross' own personal experience. There isn't a strict order to these tips, nor will everyone need to follow all of them, but they seem to answer the most common questions so many of you have.

If you suspect you have a mental health issue, you will eventually need to consult a mental health professional. Because as much as your family and friends love you, they cannot treat you. You must be under the care of someone who can properly diagnose you and prescribe a treatment plan that is right for you. We keep stressing *you* because dealing with a disorder does come down to you.

Whether your issue is severe or moderate, or even if you just want to live a more balanced life, these suggestions should help you to focus your thoughts. Your pain won't immediately vanish, and no one can promise you absolute relief. But many people have returned to normal functioning after receiving a thorough diagnosis and following a customized treatment plan.

1. Seek Help

Something is happening to you. You aren't the same person you were a couple of months ago. You don't enjoy doing anything. If you're in college, you rarely call home. If you're in high school, you avoid people at all costs. You hardly see your friends any-

What Will Happen When I Seek Help?

- You need someone who can take the intricacies of your life and make sense of them. And no, we're not talking about your roommate or your pet (though we're sure they're intuitive and supportive). You must consult an expert who can break it all down and hopefully help you figure out a better ending to the story of YOU.

- To be accurately diagnosed, you'll need to be honest and disclose your experience. How long have you had certain symptoms or episodes? How severe are they? Do other people feel that you have changed? Have you been hospitalized — if so, for how long? What other treatments have you tried, if any? What do you do when you feel out of control? How do you handle your emotions? Has there been any physical or sexual abuse in your past? Substance abuse? Is there a history of suicide in your family? Any major changes or traumas like a death, divorce, a breakup?

- Although it may feel uncomfortable to expose so much of your past, if you want to get well, you must share this information. Otherwise no one can really help or properly diagnose you. And the diagnosis is absolutely critical. It will identify what you are experiencing and why, determine your treatment plan, and help to put you on a positive course for the rest of your life. Not to be dramatic, but let's face it, the stakes are high.

- Studies have shown that the most effective form of managing a severe mental disorder is a combination of medication and therapy, but there are also other effective treatments out there that can be explored. The earlier you get a diagnosis and start treatment, the higher your chances are of being able to find the solution that works best for you and being able to lead a productive, functional life.

more. You spend most of your time sitting in your room staring at your wall. It seems like there is a piece of Styrofoam stuck between your brain and your skull, and it won't go away. Does any of this sound familiar? If so, you need to seek help.

The idea of seeking help may seem pretty simplistic (and it's obviously a large focus of this book). But still, we can't stress it enough. If you're in high school or out of college, there can be a lot of obstacles to seeking help. Maybe you (or your parents) don't have insurance. Maybe there aren't any psychologists or psychiatrists in your area. Maybe the quality of help available isn't great. Maybe you don't even know where to begin. These are all real problems, but the problems related to *not* seeking help are worse.

If you're in high school, seeking help can be a little tricky, especially if you're under 18. The first step is for you to talk to a counselor at your school. You may not want to for a whole host of reasons—the counselor is too old, doesn't get it, they'll tell my parents or kick me out of school, or I don't want anybody here at school to know about my issue. But if you're feeling bad enough to ask for help, how can it hurt to at least give your counselor a chance? You can also ask him or her if there is someone else you could be referred to. That's what they are there for. To help you. A counselor will definitely tell your parents what is happening if you are considered a threat to yourself or others. But if you're not a threat to anyone, you can ask what—if anything—the counselor must share with your parents or whomever. Every school and state may have different policies in this regard.

In most cases, you will need a parent's permission to talk to a mental health professional *other* than your school counselor. If for some reason, your parents don't want you to seek help, then you can talk to your counselor about your options. Remember, you also always have access to hotlines, websites, local mental health groups, and other resources which we have listed at the end of this book.

If you are in college, then you should know that this is one of the easiest places to seek help during your life. That doesn't mean it's entirely simple or that you won't have any complications. The counselor-to-student ratio is still 1 to 1,697, although some smaller schools have better ratios. But chances are, you already have some level of health insurance from either your college or your parents, so that's a plus. You should also have a counseling center on campus that either refers people to professionals off campus or that can possibly even help you right away. Almost all campuses offer between two to eight free visits at their counseling center. You don't need your parents' permission, but if you are going to use their insurance, then you'll want to check with your counseling center to see if the charge will show up as a visit to the wellness center or as a visit for counseling. Outside of that, no one else needs to know. If you are going to seek help, then the time is now. What are you waiting for?

Before you seek help, you should definitely educate yourself on your rights. There is a lot of apprehension out there about what can happen to information about your mental health. Know that *no one* can legally share your personal health information with other people on campus. It should all be confidential. You should not be kicked out of school unless you are considered to be a threat to yourself or others. And if that is the case, the school will be more likely to accept you again when you are healthy, if it is documented that you attempted to seek help before things got too bad. But if they have to *ask* you to leave as a result of your *not* seeking help, some schools are not as open to bringing you back.

When you approach your school's counseling center, you shouldn't have to wait weeks for an appointment, but if you do, you can ask to be referred to someone off campus. Of course, it's impossible for us to tell you the specific policies of each school in every state, so please check with your counseling center to confirm their policies.

You are taking a huge step by seeking help. If you want the best outcome, it's even better to go a step further. Educate yourself! Make sure that you know what's going on inside you, what can happen to you if you don't follow your treatment program, and lastly, know your rights. After that, you can start to work on all of the other issues. Remember, when you first start to talk about these problems, it can seem impossible to stop crying or to find the right words. It will take time, and it does get better, but not unless you begin the process and equip yourself with the emotional tools needed to build a better life. Again, the first step is just finding the courage to seek help.

Know Your Rights

Ross sits on the Leadership 21 Committee for the Bazelon Center for Mental Health Law. The committee has put together a guide to help college students understand the laws and individual rights when someone seeks help for mental health issues. To find out what you should be guaranteed in this regard, please visit www.bazelon.org.

2. Understand the Diagnosis Is Only a Starting Point

Ross has encountered thousands of people who are primarily focused on getting the right diagnosis, as they feel strongly that the diagnosis alone will immediately solve all of their problems. The diagnosis *is* critical. And to some extent, having the right diagnosis can even be empowering. It identifies what's wrong so you can learn more about yourself, trace your family's history, and maybe even meet some like-minded people who are experiencing similar things. But the diagnosis is something that needs to be kept in perspective. It's only one step in the right direction. It is by no means the end of your problems.

If anything, the diagnosis is the beginning of what for some people can be a life-long process of learning about your disorder and taking care of yourself. Think about it this way: if you tore all of the ligaments in your knee and broke your kneecap, the doctor wouldn't say: "Okay, you have no knee left. But the good news is we got the right diagnosis, so please go back out and do what you want to do! Run, swim, bike. Like I said, we got the right diagnosis. It's all downhill from here." Ridiculous, right? In reality, you would likely have to go through surgery and months of painful physical rehab before you could even use your knee again. And even after it healed, you would always run the risk of it blowing out on you.

Well, guess what? Your brain is just as much a part of your body as your knee, and when you get a diagnosis of a mental disorder, it's only a starting point for the healing process. You still need to determine what plan is going to work best for you. It could take months or years of effort to learn what is needed keep you healthy. And just like your knee, your brain can always have blowouts or relapses. Traumatic life events like the death of someone you love, a divorce, a breakup, or incidents of physical or sexual abuse can make a mental disorder resurface. And sometimes, disorders can reappear even when it seems like everything else is going fine.

Sometimes finding the right diagnosis can be extremely difficult, because certain physical conditions can cause problems that mimic some mental health issues. There is an inextricable link between your physical and mental health. So if you are having a serious problem finding a mental health diagnosis that defines your problem, you may want to get a checkup on your physical health as well, as the root of your problems could be stemming from something else.

MELANIE was diagnosed with an endocrine disorder. *For several years, every day felt like a struggle. I suffered periods of severe depression, exhaustion, and physical pain, some lasting for over a year. I had no idea what was wrong with me. Some days I'd wake only to wish that I hadn't. I felt as if I'd passed through to the other side of a mirror. I could see my old self, but had no idea how to reach her.*

After an inordinate amount of testing, my lab results revealed that I had a thyroid disease with additional endocrine complications. As I complied with my doctor's treatment program, I realized how my physical body profoundly affected my emotional health. The diagnosis freed me, but it also left me with more questions and the responsibility to find the answers. The doctor couldn't do it for me. In order to live a truly healthful life, I'd have to educate myself on the intricacies of my disease.

-----

3. Educate Yourself About Your Medication (If You Don't Like It or It Isn't Working, TELL YOUR DOCTOR)

The first visit to a psychiatrist can be intimidating. After peppering you with endless personal questions, the doctor may slap you with a diagnosis of a mental disorder. You're flooded with differing emotions—relief, confusion, denial, outrage, exhaustion—but the session isn't over. Before you leave, your doctor hands you a piece of paper, listing a psychiatric medication that you're now supposed to take to feel "normal."

You look at the psychiatrist, slowly nod, take the prescription and leave the room, reeling at the thought of having to "take meds." You might feel afraid, angry, worried, misunderstood, or you could think that you don't need the pills. Whatever the issue, taking medication is a now serious part of your treatment. And it is important to note that not everyone who visits a psychiatrist will need to receive medication. Some people will be advised to start with different forms of therapy, such as cognitive behavioral therapy or interpersonal therapy. The prescription for medication largely depends on the severity of the disorder.

If you're given medication, it is an important part of your treatment. Meds can save your life. They can also come with complications, difficulties, and major side effects, which is why it's best to research all medications. Know what you're ingesting. Few people research their psychiatric medication, taking it without knowing the side effects. Don't take that route. Empower yourself. Let your fingers do the walking and get on the internet. Talk to your doctor. Visit the library. Read the fine print on the paperwork (all medication should come with information on side effects).

This research is critical. You need to talk to your doctor and understand why a particular medication has been chosen for you, what you can expect from taking it, how long you should take it, and what you should watch out for (i.e., feeling worse than you did before the medication or other negative side effects). The process of taking medication can be a long one. You may have to take it for months or years. If you have a very severe mental disorder, you may even need medication for the rest of your life. But the earlier you start asking questions, the better off you'll be.

Monitor Yourself

Some antidepressant medications now have a black box warning on them, informing people that they should monitor their moods while taking the medication. Of course, people should be doing this with any and all medications, but especially with regard to any drugs prescribed for mental disorders. Enlist your friends, family or those close to you to help monitor you as well.

Dealing With a Mental Disorder

Medication is important, but it won't do all the work. You should also ask your doctor if there are things you can do outside of your medications to help manage your disorder. Research shows the most effective form of treatment for mental disorders is medication and therapy, but very few people know that, and even fewer actually receive both. Some people think, "If I just take my pills, then my problems will go away." However, this is not true for everyone.

Medications can be extremely effective in raising or stabilizing your mood, helping you focus, lessening anxiety, or reducing psychotic symptoms. Some people will respond to medication right away and be able to function the way they used to. Others may need to try different combinations over a period of years before they discover what is most effective. And still others may never find the perfect medications to help them. But no matter what the situation, the meds are there to help you in various ways, so that you can work on other parts of your disorder.

If a woman took blood pressure pills for her heart, then continued to drink alcohol, smoke cigarettes, not exercise, eat crappy food, and she didn't do anything to help beyond taking medication, then she would run the risk of dying a lot sooner. If you or anyone you know is taking medication for a problem with the brain and you don't talk about it, you don't work on it, or worse—you drink, do drugs, or hurt yourself—then you are not going to deal with the disorder nearly as well as you could.

Sometimes people like to go off of their medication. They may worry about side effects. They may feel like their meds aren't working. But medications don't always start to work instantly. The transition period—from when you start taking your medicine to when it actually starts working—can feel like hell. Sometimes you may not know if you are coming or going. But if you stick with it, you'll be likely to see an improvement.

Other people may actually like some of the feelings associated with their disorders. For example, some people who have bipolar disorder enjoy the feelings of invincibility associated with their manic highs. But going on and off medications, or not sticking with your treatment, is just going to make things worse. It may seem easier to go back to old coping mechanisms like getting drunk or high, but in doing so, you will be delaying the medication's progress. If you have serious issues, and if your doctor thinks medication could help, then it's in your best interest to consider his or her advice and comply with your treatment plan. Remember, you sought help in the first place because the way things were wasn't working for you. The meds are there to make things better—if you give them a chance to work properly.

If you've given your medication a chance and you truly think it's not working, then you must talk to your doctor before quitting "cold turkey." The body is extremely sensitive. When you suddenly stop any psychiatric medication, you can cause unwanted changes to your body. Your doctor is well aware of these risks and can wean you off any medication that's not right for you. You might have the wrong dose, or maybe it's the wrong medication altogether. But you certainly won't find an answer if you keep your feelings to yourself—and your doctor in the dark.

You may think you don't need meds. You may worry they'll change you somehow—make you worse, alter your personality, make you exhausted, hyper, or gain weight. The truth is, they *may* change you. Not necessarily in these particular ways, but everyone responds to medicine differently. Not all medications are the same. There are different families of medications with different potential for certain side effects. You may need to experiment to find the one that works for you.

There are many people who greatly benefit from taking medication. You could be one of them. If you feel resistance to the idea, think about what's holding you back. Is it fear, shame, judgment? Whatever it is, is it important enough to make you risk your life? Some medications have saved people's lives—they could even save yours.

This is too important not to say again: *if you're unhappy with your medication for any reason, tell your psychiatrist or doctor.* If they don't seem to care or respond to your satisfaction, then find another psychiatrist or doctor who does.

4. Learn About Your Disorder— Adjust Your Lifestyle

Educating yourself on your disorder is critical in order to have a healthy recovery. You can do this by reading books, going to group sessions to meet other people, researching the disorder online, possibly getting into web chats, and talking about how the disorder affects you. All of these are hugely important steps to take and cannot be stressed enough. The less you know about your condition, the more other people can take advantage of you or exploit your lack of knowledge. *You need to be your own best advocate.*

Alternative Treatments

You have a lot of options when seeking help. We just discussed medication, but here are some alternative treatments that have also been proven successful for some people, sometimes in combination with medication: psychotherapy, behavior therapy, psychoanalysis, cognitive therapy, family therapy, movement/art/music therapy, group therapy, electric convulsive treatment, self-help, diet and nutrition, pastoral counseling, animal assisted therapies, culturally-based healing arts like acupuncture, ayurveda, yoga/meditation, Native American traditional practices, stress reduction techniques like biofeedback, guided imagery or visualization, massage therapy. There are also new technology-based applications like telemedicine, telephone counseling, electronic communications, radio psychiatry, and lastly some ideas that focus on mental wellness like psychodrama, hypnotherapy, recreational, and Outward Bound-type nature programs. There is a lot of information available on these various treatments. You can also ask your mental health counselor, therapist or doctor about them as well.

COLLEEN was diagnosed with anxiety, depression, anorexia and bulimia. It took years for her to learn the best way to manage her disorders. *One thing I have going for me is that I LOVE to learn. I read and talk and listen all the time. Reading about other's experiences, talking to people that go through mental disorders on any level, helps me feel that I am not alone. It also helps me to understand what things work well for others and test it out on myself. Yoga, for example, works really well for my dad and best friend who both struggle with mild depression. I began this practice this year, and it really helps me, too. Working out and eating well in moderation also helps. I am currently in the process of discovery, and I am finding that it may be more helpful for me to be at home—around a lot of support—frequently, if not permanently.*

As Colleen points out, learning is a large part of this process and taking action is the next part. Gathering knowledge about what you are experiencing is an awesome starting point, but once you start to learn, then you have to make those lifestyle changes that will help to keep your educational process going.

When you're in high school, you're probably living at home with your family. Maybe they keep an eye on your treatment and are able to help you manage. Or if you are closer to your friends and feel more comfortable talking to them, they can help out. But what happens when you have a really great treatment program that is working at home, and then you go away to college?

Perhaps the most common mistake young people make when they go to college with a mental disorder is not having a plan. Maybe they see college as a place to start over, move on, meet new people who don't know about their issues. They relax and slack off on whatever treatment or behavior had been previously working for them. But in fact, college—or any time you're facing a big change in your routine—is when you most *need* to have a plan in place for dealing with your mental disorder.

ROSS *While I was in my second semester back at American University and wanted to make these positive changes in my life, I felt I had the education. I had been learning about bipolar disorder for eleven years, since first seeing my brother go through it. I could give a dissertation on what the disorder was, but couldn't give you even one sentence on how to deal with it. The first thing I needed to do was create a time-managed structure for my life. I needed to get regulated amounts of sleep. I started to try to go to bed at the same time every night and wake up at the same time every morning. In the beginning this was hard, because some nights I was tired, and some nights I wasn't. To counter that, I started exercising every day to make sure that I would be tired enough to sleep. Exercise soon became a regular activity for me. I also had the rest of my day structured around work and classes. I would know exactly when I could read for my classes each night, or in between classes and work. I budgeted time for writing papers and seeing friends.*

Sometimes other parts of your life can suffer when you set up a structure. Ross didn't have much of a social life when he went back to American University, although he did have close friends and a girlfriend whom he would see regularly. In some ways, he felt he had imprisoned himself in order to find the structure that was vital for him to survive. But ultimately, it worked. He went on to graduate cum laude from American University.

The key to making changes that will work for you is to remember that everyone is different, and everyone has different needs. But clearly *some* kind of lifestyle change is necessary, or you wouldn't be looking for help. Again—the more you know about your disorder, the more realistic adjustments you will be able to make.

5. Cooperate With Your Mental Health Professional

Once you find the right diagnosis and a mental health professional whom you trust, it's important to try as hard as you can to cooperate with your psychiatrist or psychologist and stick with whatever treatment he or she sets up for you. Sometimes you may try to dodge your treatment by convincing yourself that things really aren't that bad. But maybe you don't even know how bad they can be. You want to keep going through the motions and keep trying to make everything okay, but at some point your disorder *will* catch up to you.

You can only hide for so long. Eventually, you may hit rock bottom, and you will no longer be able to deny that your life has spun out of control. But here's the thing: everyone's "rock bottom" is different. Some people crash so hard they actually hit the grave; they have a fatal accident, or they take their own lives. While others are moved to turn their lives

How Can I Plan My Life at College if I Have a Mental Disorder?

- Make it a priority to go to the counseling center as soon as you get to campus to start scheduling appointments and learning about what they offer.

- If your counseling center can only see you for a certain period of time, find out what your options are, how many visits you get, and what you can do to supplement those visits.

- Know where you can get your medications.

- Talk to the mental health professional you've been seeing back home, and find out how you can contact him or her if you need to.

- Find resources in the surrounding community if the counseling center can't help you.

- Call your insurance company and ask them what they cover and don't cover.

- Most importantly, prepare yourself for change. College is a big transition for any student, so be aware that change can trigger a relapse or cause you to have difficulty adjusting to your treatment.

- Recognize your warning signs and adjust your lifestyle accordingly.

- If you have to leave college at any point to deal with your disorder, know that it is okay. You can return later, or you may choose to take another life path. But having to leave school for a while is not necessarily the end of the road.

around. It's important to find some inspiration to do something about your life *before* you're out of options—and whatever that something is, it's just as important that you stick to it. Identifying the problem is only half the battle. You must be involved with your treatment.

Being involved with your treatment means taking your medications, being honest in therapy, working on what is identified in therapy, and cooperating with your doctors to find what plan works best for you. It also means that you cannot binge drink, do drugs, lie to or hide things from your mental health professional, not sleep, have endless sexual escapades, eat unhealthily, and not take care of yourself. *Your treatment will not be effective* if you behave this way. If you do any of those things while taking your meds or just go through the motions of therapy without putting in hard work, you will not see improvement. And in that case, it is not the meds' fault that they don't work—nor is it your therapist's fault that he or she couldn't take away your problems. You have to participate in your own recovery.

We know it can be hard to be that one guy or that one girl at a party who isn't drinking—because you have a mental health issue, or especially if you're on meds. Some people might nurse one drink the whole night, while others are open about the fact that they simply are not going to drink. It can be a challenge no matter what you do, but in the long run you should try as hard as you can to either feel comfortable without having to drink heavily, or finding social activities that don't include alcohol. They do exist! (And remember, your health is always more important than some party.)

It's Not A Competition!

Finding the right treatment for a mental disorder is not a competition. Sometimes young people will hear what worked for their friends and want to try that same treatment. Other times students will be upset that a friend or someone else with same disorder is doing better than they are, because they still haven't found a treatment plan that works. We can't stress enough that your disorder is unique to you. So you must find what works best for you. Don't be discouraged by other people who seem to be doing better than you are. Just focus as hard as you can on your own treatment. It may take weeks, months, or years to find something that works well for you, but feeling bad because other people are doing better won't help. You can't change your biology, but you can change how you deal with it. Stay focused on what you can do.

6. Develop Friendships with People Other than Your Therapist

ALISON's brother took his own life. *Once Brian did seek help, his life was somewhat ruled by his mental health care. He came home from Columbia University during his sophomore year and started seeing a psy-*

chiatrist near our home several days a week, for both talk therapy and medication. He underwent 16 long months of experimenting with treatments—different medications, different frequencies of doctor visits, different activities. At the same time, however, he masked his thoughts and feelings from everyone around him, except for my mom and his doctor. So he essentially had no peer support—like me or his friends—to help him through his illness. As such a talented young man, one of Brian's biggest struggles was with reconciling what he had always dreamed for himself and what his new life with a mental disorder had become. Without any positive role models to look up to, Brian convinced himself that this struggle would become a lifelong one, and that he would never again be the successful person that he once was.

Because you and your therapist discuss really intimate things, you may feel that he or she is a friend. Okay, a paid friend, but still, a friend. And it's great that you can talk to your therapist about your innermost thoughts and feelings. But it's also really important to have a support group of friends—or even just one close friend—who you can talk to about these issues. It can take a long time for you to be able to talk about anything deep in your life. It's hard to open up to other people about emotions, and you may be afraid. But talking to a friend, family member, partner, or someone you see on a regular basis outside of your therapist can really help you to feel better when you are in therapy.

The Psych Ward

Your disorder may be severe enough to require a stay in a psychiatric ward. This can cause some people a lot of anxiety, stress and fear. However, psychiatric wards and rehabilitation centers are set up to help you. When people get sick from pneumonia or something severe, they need to go to a hospital. Sometimes our disorders get so severe that we must go to a hospital to get stabilized.

If you go to a psychiatric ward or rehab center you can expect nurses or even doctors to regularly monitor your treatments. They will give you your medication at the times it is needed. They may take blood samples to test the levels of the medications in your body. You will have certain times where you are expected to sleep. You will also have to be involved in group activities, like painting, making things, or therapy sessions. When you arrive you will be told what privileges you may have: phone calls, visitors, computers, possible trips out of the hospital, or watching television. Some people may have more strict limits because of their disorders and triggers.

If you're hospitalized for attempting to take your own life, you'll be placed on some type of suicide watch, which may include someone having to have eyes on you at all times, even when you sleep. You will also have any materials or objects with which you could harm yourself taken away. You may have to shower

---

with the door open. They will monitor you to see when your thoughts of suicide are lessened to determine when some of these restrictions can be lifted.

Please view your stay in any hospital as a chance for you to take some much-needed time to deal with your disorder. The more honest you are and the more you work on finding what out exactly what works best for you, the better off you will be when you leave.

ROSS *My therapist could ask great questions, or put me in situations where I had to think about what was going on. And some days I would feel comfortable talking, but a lot of times what I was revealing was so new to me that I didn't know how to expand any more about it. I started to talk to my best friend and my girlfriend at the time about some of what we had discussed in therapy. Being that they ultimately knew me better than my therapist did, they could help me fill in some of the blanks. For example, my therapist identified that some of my self-hatred came from when my brother left the family, but my therapist didn't know my brother. So talking to people who did know him helped to make me feel more comfortable when talking to my therapist.*

In later chapters, we'll talk more specifically about the roles of friends and relationships, as well as some of the ways in which you may be able to start talking to those close to you about these issues. If you are able to start this process, it can only help you. However, it should only be with people you trust—people who are close to you—people who truly care about you.

7. You Are NOT Your Disorder

We hear it all the time. "*I'm* bipolar." "*I'm* ADD." "*I'm* ADHD." "*I'm* anorexic." "*I'm* schizophrenic or bulimic." Some people proclaim their disorder as if that is their only identity. And it makes sense in certain situations, but you should definitely be careful about your choice of words. *No disorder—no matter what it is—defines you.* The name of your disorder may sound severe, damaging, daunting, or even controlling. But it doesn't have to define your whole life.

The problem with people saying, "*I'm* (fill in disorder)" is that they are identifying themselves by their disorder, and not their whole selves. Have you ever noticed how people with a physical illness, like cancer, don't say, "*I am* breast cancer"? You don't hear people say, "*I am* AIDS." People with diabetes say, "I have diabetes" or "I am a diabetic," not "*I'm* diabetes." It's much healthier to say, "My name is (your name here) and I *have* bipolar disorder," than it is to say, "*I'm* bipolar."

The reason this distinction is important is because it casts a more positive outlook on your treatment. You'll start to think of your disorder as something you can manage, not simply something you're stuck with, or something that can't be helped. You should never go home, freak out on your boyfriend or girlfriend, and then excuse it by saying "Hey, I'm bipolar, babe, deal with it." If something like that happens, a better approach would be, "Wow, I really flipped out there. I feel badly about that. What can I do to keep that from happening again? What happened just before my freak out? Was it something I thought or felt? Did I feel scared, insecure or angry? If so, why? Did I overreact to something you said?"

These are just some of the questions you can ask yourself to better understand what triggers you. If you had cancer, you would want to know the risks or what you can do to improve your health. It's the same with your heart or other injured body parts. Certainly this process is more challenging when you are dealing with the brain and your emotions, but it's critical if you want to take responsibility for your life.

You didn't choose to have a mental disorder. You didn't choose to go through extremely difficult experiences. However, you *can* make the choice to deal with your disorder healthily and responsibly, no matter how long that takes.

8. Maintenance

A lot of people in the mental health field use the word "recovery." But what does that word means with regard to a mental disorder? Think about it: you recover from a broken leg, and you can walk again. You recover from the flu and can go back to school. You recover from an extreme episode with a mental disorder and can function again. But what now? Are you in constant recovery? Are you a recovering bipolar person? Will it ever end?

Maintaining your mental health is a lifelong process. If you have a diagnosed disorder, and if you want to be truly functional, you need to enter a deeper process of understanding your disorder. Many healthcare professionals call this process "maintenance."

Even if you never have another episode or experience with a mental disorder for the rest of your life, there are steps you'll need to take to ensure your ongoing health. For instance, you'll need to recognize your warning signs, continue to educate yourself, read relevant books and materials, and stay up to date on your treatment. It's a long process, and it's never really over. Whether your disorder was severe or not so severe, you'll need to be aware of the possibility of it returning, and you'll need to maintain whatever treatment works best for you. So "maintenance" can be a good descriptive term for the process; it almost makes more sense than "recovery."

Maintenance, much like the other issues we discussed in this chapter, is not easy and requires a lot of work. For maintenance to even begin, you have to already be in a pretty good place with your disorder. For example:

- If you had a severe episode, you need to have recovered from it.

- You're seeing mental health professionals you trust.

- You discovered a treatment plan that works.

- You've had time to reflect on your disorder.

- You can recognize your warning signs and triggers. You're aware of your emotions and how certain stresses in your life can bring about negative episodes.

- You continue to educate yourself on your disorder.

- You have healthy friendships and relationships to support you.

- You have the ability to make healthy decisions.

Dealing With a Mental Disorder

ROSS *In the beginning, the hardest thing about maintenance for me was being able to stick with it. I remember I was doing well for about two months. I hadn't been drinking or partying and was doing okay. Then one night, someone shoved a bottle of Jack Daniels in my face and the next thing I knew, I had cheated on my girlfriend and couldn't remember driving home. Obviously, I woke up the next day feeling terrible.*

All of the feelings of self-hatred came back. I told myself that this is who I would always be. I was extremely lucky to be able to call my friends—and even my girlfriend—and tell them what happened. With their support, I realized that I couldn't let the two months of positive work just slip away after one negative episode. I couldn't let that one mistake define me and my recovery. I had to continue to take the things I had learned from the previous two months—and most importantly that night— and try my best not to let it happen again. That day I was able to recognize some of my triggers.

Today, while I haven't had a crippling episode with bipolar disorder for close to eight years, I still hallucinate sometimes. I still have mini-episodes. I have extreme anger at times, moods I can't control, and I even still have thoughts of death and thoughts of killing myself, sometimes. To some extent, this disorder is going to be part of me forever. However, I am also more able to talk about what I am going through with the people closest to me, and they are also good at identifying whenever I might not be "okay" I work hard to identify any and all warning signs and symptoms. I know now that

I am more at risk during times of change, loss, or whenever I'm stressed. So if I am going through something difficult, I try to stay far away from alcohol or any hint of it. I have been able to make a lot of changes like that over the years.

My life was so ridiculously structured in college that as I moved forward it became a bit unhealthy for me, because I was keeping myself from social situations or other things I normally enjoyed to make sure I was okay. Obviously, after missing out on so many things, I didn't want to go down a slippery slope and lose it all again. However, with the love and support of my present girlfriend, I have been able to put myself in those situations I was hiding from, which is much healthier for me in the long run. It's hard to come out of the box I had created to help myself survive. But as I get older and am able to better recognize things about myself, it is also healthy for me to experience new things so I can continue to learn to adapt. The structured existence I had created did let me function the best way I could at the time, but it also limited me in a way that wouldn't continue to be healthy forever.

Structure can be an excellent tool for helping someone to regain a sense of normalcy, especially after experiencing a severe mental disorder. At the same time, structure can hinder you if it's taken too far. If you have a treatment program in place and want to change something about it, you should always discuss it with a mental health professional.

You may have a great idea for your treatment plan that could really work for you, but it's critical to run it by someone who understands your mental disorder and your potential blind spots. Think about driving a car. You can see the road and the cars around you, but there are still a few angles that you can't see clearly. Sometimes mental disorders can give you a similar perspective on your life. If you move in those directions, you could set yourself up for a crash. That's why it's good to run things by somebody who may be able to see those things you can't.

Hope Is On The Way

All of these suggestions can help you and your loved ones to better understand and deal with your disorder. They can also give you hope. But they are only a starting point, and listed in no specific order. Each one can help you in different ways. They may not come together all at once, they may not come easily, or they may not come at all. You may discover them at different phases of your maintenance program, or you may find some of your own that aren't included here. Everyone's path is different. There are no rules—only lessons, and the steps you'll take towards regaining your health.

What Can I Do To Help Myself?

Dr. Richard Kadison in his book, *College of the Overwhelmed*, offers these tips to help you prevent certain mental health issues you already have—or may be likely to get—from occurring. These are helpful ways to deal with a mental disorder while you are in college—but they work well in high school, too.

(more)

What Can I Do To Help Myself? (cont.)

- **Exercise often.** Dr. Kadison says the benefits of exercise are to improve alertness, give you increased energy, stimulate the immune system, and keep off excess weight. He recommends little things like taking a longer walk to class, using the stairs, or taking study breaks to raise your heart rate.

- **Eat well.** Dr. Kadison knows about the "freshman fifteen!" He recommends drinking a lot of water, adding a salad to each meal, substituting a piece of fruit for a dessert each day, substituting whole wheat bread for white bread, having a bowl of fortified cereal instead of a bagel, and eating a vegetable at each meal. Try not to keep high calorie snacks (like potato chips) in your dorm room.

- **Sleep well.** Dr. Kadison says the idea that students who stay up all night to study get better GPAs is a myth. It is actually the students who get a good night's sleep who get the best grades. Less than six hours of sleep a night can lead to deficits in attention, concentration, memory, and critical thinking. It can contribute to depression, irritability, and anxiety. To get better sleep, he advises staying away from caffeine, nicotine, and alcohol in the late afternoon or evening. (Cigarettes or soda can make it difficult to sleep, and alcohol will likely disrupt your sleep after you drop off.) Don't nap during the day if you're having trouble falling asleep at night, and don't exercise right before bedtime. Instead, develop a nighttime ritual such as relaxing for 15 to 30 minutes before you sleep. If you can't sleep, don't toss and turn worrying about not sleeping. Just get out of bed and read or do something relaxing until you are tired enough to fall asleep.

- **Stay connected.** Check in regularly with your family or the people who supported you most before you went away to college. If you lose contact for a month or more, it can be hard to go back. And if you start having a problem, it can be good to keep that communication open. Part of being mature is learning when to share problems and concerns and when to ask for help. Also, stay connected to your friends, and develop new friendships at college.

- **Organize and evaluate your time.** Use time management to be more productive. Block out time periods. Allocate the time for work or social activities. You can use a daily planner, Palm Pilot, or anything to make a schedule. This will help you manage and balance your time more effectively. You'll have more time for your relationships, as well as your physical and mental health.

- **Reach out.** You are in a diverse environment, so take the time to learn about different people, different cultures, and different ways of life. Accepting people who look and act differently from you is a great stress reducer. Many people fear things that deviate from their own sense of normalcy. They shut down when they are faced with someone—or something—that doesn't feel comfortable or familiar. If you can relate to this, then make an extra effort to learn about new people, cultures, and ways of life that are different from your own. When you accept people who challenge your comfort levels, you reduce your stress levels and grow as a person.

- **Be informed.** Know the signs and symptoms of trouble. Pay attention to yourself, your needs, and your feelings. Be proactive about getting information. Be on the lookout for informational sessions on campus that are relevant for you, and for other chances to further educate yourself.

- **Don't suffer long. Don't suffer alone.** If you recognize that you aren't doing well, talk to someone about it and seek help right away. Dr. Kadison says the patterns and behaviors practiced in college don't disappear when you graduate, so it's best to address them now.

CHAPTER 5

THE "F" WORD:
Families

"Everybody pretend to be normal!"
—Little Miss Sunshine
(Fox Searchlight, 2006)

ROSS *That night, we had just won a basketball game, and afterwards I went to Friendly's with all my friends to celebrate, just like we always did. I had already been wrestling with thoughts of death and suicide for about three months, but for some reason, it was on that ride home that I decided to finally end my pain and do it. I stared out the window in the backseat and looked at the crisp winter ground. The farmlands that were so familiar to me as a child seemed so distant, lit by the moonlight. I thanked the guys who drove* *me home and opened the door for what I thought would be the last time.*

I went upstairs to my bedroom. In one last attempt to stop myself, I lay paralyzed by my bedroom phone. The anguish of depression tightened every muscle in my body until I was in a fetal position, barely able to call a friend. And when I finally did call, I had no words. My throat was choked off by the agony of my thoughts. I hung up. I walked across the hallway to my bathroom to end it. But before anything too major happened my dad walked by. He wasn't supposed to be home. But he was, and he stopped and asked me what I was doing.

I froze. I shook. My family had never talked about emotion. My oldest brother had left the family when I was 16, and I didn't get along with my middle brother at all. So I had no idea how to tell my dad what I was thinking in that moment. He asked me to come downstairs to talk to him. I walked into the kitchen, and told him that if he didn't take me to the hospital, I was going to kill myself. Just then, the phone rang. It turns out that the call I had made earlier wasn't entirely audible, but the person on the other end had heard something, and suspected that something bad may have happened. My parents panicked. Of course they didn't want to believe I really wanted to die. Then they made a phone call. I just didn't want to be there at all anymore.

My parents cried all the way to the hospital. In the curtained area of the waiting room, I was briefly left alone and ended up hurting myself. The nurses and doctors wrestled with me, then gave me a tranquilizer so they could admit me to the psychiatric ward. After I was admitted, my parents came to visit every chance they could. My brother Vance came too.

I went on to graduate from high school and attend American University. The adjustment didn't go well for me, though. I ultimately had a major relapse with bipolar disorder. One day, I threw a guy onto the floor at the pharmacy where I was waiting for my new meds. The next day, I pushed someone down an escalator. It was on that day that I called my dad to come get me, and I took a medical leave of absence from school.

I was hospitalized again. When I got out of the hospital I weighed 230 pounds, which was about 60 pounds more than I weighed when I'd started college. I felt hopeless—like I had nothing to live for. But my parents helped me get a job. They asked me to enroll in community college and tried to get me to function a little bit. I returned to American University four years after I started, and when I finally graduated, my parents were there to watch me walk across the stage in my cap and gown.

The support I received from my parents was a huge help. They let me live at their house the entire time I wasn't in Washington, DC. They didn't always know what to do or say, but they were there. They loved me and my two brothers as much or even more than any parents ever could, but they really didn't know exactly what to do. My mom was raised in a home where issues like this were just swept under the rug. You didn't talk about them. My dad grew up with an alcoholic father who never touched him, never hugged him, never said "I love you." He couldn't have friends over because he never knew what state his dad would be in when he came home. We have depression, bipolar disorder, alcoholism, and anxiety on both sides of my family, but no one ever really talked openly about it.

I can honestly say that my parents raised me the best way they knew how, but again—I needed more help than they could give me in order to deal with these issues. I had birthday parties, new clothes, rides to every practice imaginable, but I never had the words or any sense of comfort when I would try to talk about emotion or bipolar disorder. And for that reason, my parents became the enemy for a time. They were the ones I would want to blame and the ones I would take everything out on. Our house was filled with anger and rage, especially unfairly toward my mom. I don't know if it was because I expected them to take away my pain, or that the disorder just had me so much on edge that I snapped. I can't stress enough how much my parents cared, but they didn't always know what to do. And for the longest time, caring just didn't cut it.

Families and Mental Health

From the moment you open your eyes, whether you're adopted or not, your family is yours for life. There are no exchanges or returns—at least not in the formative years. Families are like living organisms. They take on a life of their own, and regardless of how we may feel about it, we're bound to them until the day we die. They define us, shape our identity, and determine how we feel about ourselves in the world. Families can be your greatest source of inspiration, or the main cause of your most unthinkable pain. Or sometimes, they represent a little of both.

As a young adult, you may have tried to distance yourself from your family in order to establish an identity all your own. Not to bore you with developmental psychology, but this is a normal part of growing up. Everyone does this in his or her own way, and some more than others. But no matter how far you stray, your family can help you regress back to that infant state, the feeling of your most simple and basic self.

Obviously, mental disorders will complicate a family. They can cause a family to fall apart. They can cause generations of unresolved pain, suffering, confusion, and dysfunction, leading to extreme cases of insecurity, lack of trust, and fear of commitment. Conversely, the discovery of a mental disorder can also heal a family that was once splintered. Love can heal trauma. Its powers are profound. If given the opportunity, it can even bring someone back from the brink.

If you're reading this and have a mental disorder, you know how complicated it can make things for your family. And the flip side is true also—if your family member has a disorder, you can't escape dealing with it yourself. Let's look at what can happen to a family when one of its members has a mental disorder.

When Parents Don't Know What to Do

Parents deal with mental disorders in a variety of ways. Some parents are supportive and do everything they can to help their children. Others become ultra protective and fearful of any changes or problems. Some never address the issue—not because they don't care, but because they don't know where to begin. They feel utterly powerless and ineffective, like they might end up causing even more problems for their kids. Can you imagine what this must feel like? You love someone more than you can even describe in words. They're a part of you.

Yet you can't reach that person emotionally or help him or her get better. It would suck to be a parent in this situation. And being a kid dealing with a frustrated parent is no picnic. Let's face it; it's tough for everyone involved.

MARC describes a depressive episode **that struck when he was 23.** *I finally made the phone call to my parents, articulating to them in my angst-ridden state that due to my depression I had been rendered helpless. I told them about the previous several weeks and how I had no desire to even leave my bed. My father suggested that he travel to DC to accompany me back home to Los Angeles. With his help, I wouldn't have to think. Like most children, I have a vivid image of being taken to college by one of my parents, left to start a new chapter of my life. Once again, one of my parents would be present on another journey, this time on a voyage no one really wanted to take. My father was now taking me home…because I could not get there on my own.*

There are a lot of homes where the parents may care, but yet they don't know how to talk about feelings. Maybe they don't know how to deal with mental health issues. In that case, *you* can be the one to open that communication. Let parents know what you need and what they can do to help you.

Or maybe you've tried communicating, and it doesn't work. In that case, you may need to accept that your parents are probably never going to change. They may be the same for as long as you live, simply because that it's the way they were raised. As hard as this can be to understand, it may be the reality you are facing. And let's be honest: it's frustrating to never really be known or understood emotionally. But on a lot of levels, it's better than having parents who don't care at all. Even if all your parents can offer you is a roof over your head, it's still better than having to live on the street. That may be terrible to hear, but it's true. And because your parents *do* care, know that there is room for change—if not now, perhaps in the future.

When you're living at home, some parents are torn between pushing you to get out, and coddling you to make sure nothing bad ever happens. Should they take care of everything for you, so you don't have to worry? Should they pressure you to do things that you don't want to do—find a job, go back to school? Talking to a professional is sometimes the best way for them to figure out how best to help you. Mental disorders are complicated. You won't just wake up one morning and find your disorder is gone. But by learning more about it and trying to do as many things as you can to improve—even on the worst days, you can make progress—and your parents can help you. The more they know about the disorder themselves, the better they'll know what to do.

The best thing for parents to do is to offer you support, but without trying to protect you from everything. One of the most important things that Ross's parents did for him, which may not even have been intentional, is to help empower him to see that he was more than just his disorder. They worked hard to help him find a job and go back to school. They encouraged him to work on getting better.

> ## Empowering vs. Enabling
>
> When a family member is trying to help someone with a disorder, there's a fine line between **empowering** and **enabling**. When someone gets out of the hospital, has to leave school, or is diagnosed with a disorder, it can be a natural reaction to try do everything for that person and greatly limit her responsibility. In some cases, this may be necessary, at least temporarily. However, at some point it is important to help the person focus on things she is capable of and empower her to work on finding ways to cope with life. Not everyone may be capable of this, and there are different time-tables for each person, but empowerment is a step in the right direction. When people with disorders have everything done for them, it just enables their dependency and lack of ability, making it hard for them to change. The best way to work on walking this line is to consult with a mental health professional.

Ross' relationship with his parents changed when he was able to start verbalizing what he needed from them. And because they cared, they tried their best to make certain changes. No one wanted every interaction to be filled with anger, so they all worked on their communication. It took them several years to figure that out, and even when they were communicating better, his oldest brother Thad still hadn't spoken to anyone in the family for nearly seven years.

With all that the family had been through together, Ross felt a deep need to reconnect with Thad, so he tracked him down on the Internet and emailed him. He wasn't sure if Thad would even answer, but within a few hours, Ross received a response. Ross cried when he saw his brother's name appear on his computer screen. It had been seven years since they'd communicated at all. Thad admitted to missing the family. Ross and his middle brother, Vance, reconnected with their brother slowly, catching up on those missing years. A couple of months after the first contact, they all met up in New York City. Shortly after that meeting, Thad spoke to their mom and dad. Ultimately, this led to Ross bringing Thad home for the first time in nearly a decade. Today, their family continues to grow closer.

ROSS *I think it takes a family to bring a family back together. Sure, I reached out to Thad, but he was willing to admit what points he needed to deal with and my parents were also willing to change, within their limits. Today, my brothers and I talk to each other about our emotions, but I still rarely talk about that with my parents. They are parents. When I do talk about emotion, they tend to want to try to fix it.*

I know who I can go to when I have problems with my disorder. I never went to my parents with my emotions before and I don't really do it now. I have people in my life who can offer that sort of help. However, I know I have my parents' support—I know they will be there for me—no matter what. When Thad decided to move from Florida to California, it was my parents who flew down to pack him up and drive him across country. And it is our parents who will always be there to welcome us home. Without these disorders, I don't know if my family would have become so disjointed, but I also don't know if we would have been able to come back together, either.

Ross was lucky. Really lucky. In the end, his whole family was committed to working out their differences. Every family has to be willing to admit faults, know when to listen, when to shut up, and what to do to work things out. It isn't easy, and there's no quick fix. And sometimes, it's anything but fun. But it can work.

If you know that your parents love and care about you but don't know what to say or do, there are a number of things you can try. You can try to educate them as much as you can about your disorder and communicate what you like and don't like, or what you need and don't need from them. Communication is absolutely vital. If you don't tell them how you feel, then they won't be able to truly understand you. Talking with a mental health professional will also help you learn ways to express yourself when dealing with your parents. If you don't think they will respond to you, it can also help to have a friend of the family—or someone they trust—approach them instead. But be careful with that one, because these issues can be embarrassing. You don't want to make it more uncomfortable by bringing in someone they don't know.

If You're On Your Own

Ross had parents who were there for him. Granted, they didn't know exactly what to do or say, but they tried to do whatever they could. Sometimes you're dealing with a mental disorder and your parents *don't* care. They may not ever fully believe that you have a problem. They could try to block you from treatment or ostracize you because you made a decision to seek help. Or you may be in a situation where your parents are plagued by their own problems or disorders, and as a result, have no real capacity to help you.

MARTHA suffers from depression and grew up with a mother who has schizophrenia and a father who is an alcoholic. When she was 16 she decided to run away. *Living in a four-room apartment doesn't leave much space for avoidance and often my dad would corner me in my room, blocking the door, and invade my privacy by standing there for what could be a half hour or more talking to me about his problems and intimate feelings. One particular day, this got to be too unbearable for me and I tried to leave the apartment. My dad and I ended up fighting. He threw me up against the wall, and I then took off, running out the front door.*

I escaped to a friend's house, and returned home later when I felt a little calmer. I went directly into my room and decided I would leave for good. I left a note for my sister, packed some clothes and climbed out of my bedroom window. I stayed at a friend's house and called my mom in the morning, but never went home again. I searched for a while before finding someone who would allow me to stay with their family. I stayed at my friend's house until I graduated from high school and went away to college. It wasn't easy. I had to deal with some resentment and hard times with the family I was living with, but I felt it was best to be away from the dysfunction in my home. I stayed in touch with my sister and spoke to my mom occasionally. But I avoided speaking to my father at all costs. I only saw him when I was required to have him sign papers or certain legal things. From age 17 to 19 I felt the situation at home got even more difficult for my sister and mother. At one point, I had to get a restraining order placed against my father in an attempt to protect my mother and sister. The combination of my mother's schizophrenia and father's alcoholism created a severely toxic environment.

My mother had another episode and I felt that if she went back home to my dad that the cycle would just continue, so I called my grandparents and my uncle and arranged for her to go down there for a "vacation." She divorced my father a few years later. My father did not put up a fight about her leaving. I was just happy that she was out of that horrible and hazardous environment. She hasn't had nearly as many episodes since she left, and I truly do believe that her stressful interactions with my father had a lot to do with her needing to "escape" the conscious world at times by stopping her meds and relapsing into her schizophrenia.

Martha had been dealing with bouts of depression since she was a child. At age 20 she had a major episode of depression, and she's always had to deal with her depression without her family. She's never told them she has the disorder or asked for their help.

Martha discovered at a young age that if her parents felt anything negative was happening to her, she would be punished physically or have certain things taken away. Or her parents simply wouldn't be able to cope with it, reacting with anxiety, fear, or anger. Because of their disorders, Martha was never supposed to have problems. Instead, she was the designated caretaker who needed to have it together at all times.

If you are in Martha's situation, with no support from within your home, then you may need to follow her example. If your family is not there to support you, it's important to remember that you still deserve to have people in your life who care about you and want to help you. You'll just have to look harder for them.

- **Friends.** Find friends who will be close to you, support you, and not leave at the first sign of trouble (like when you have a bad day). True friends can help fill the hole left by your family.

- **Support groups.** Another great way to have understanding and support are open support groups. They can help you identify certain problems in your life, while also making connections to other like-minded people.

- **Mental health professionals.** You may have no one in your personal life you feel you can talk to. So it may have to come down to a conversation between just you and your psychologist, therapist, doctor, psychiatrist, or other professional. And this is okay. You may feel somewhat isolated at first, but as you work through your issues, you may find it easier to make and maintain stronger and more meaningful friendships in the future.

- **Education.** Books, websites, brochures, or anything about your disorder can help you better understand what is happening to you and what you can do about it.

- **Spirituality.** A belief in something larger than yourself—whether it is your religion, faith, or just an overall connection to humanity–can help.

- **Music.** A lot of people find music to be a release when they don't have the words, the time, or just don't know what to say or do. However, be careful in your choice of music—it can help you release a lot of emotions, but for some people, particular kinds of music can actually serve to reinforce negative feelings.

- **Healthy lifestyle choices.** This may be the most important component when trying to break out of the damage your family dynamic created.

It may never be possible to open a relationship with your parents or get them to understand your problems. This lack of understanding can feel like rejection and can hurt more than anything in the world. But remember, you don't need to give up, either. You can try to approach your parents using some of the other advice from this chapter. If you're loving and persistent, you may help them identify their own issues, which could help to bring you all closer.

While Martha doesn't regularly speak to her father anymore, she has always kept in touch with her mother and nurtured a relationship with her years after her parents' divorce.

MARTHA suffers from depression and grew up with a mother who has schizophrenia and a father who suffers from alcoholism. *I think what helped heal the disconnect between my mom and me was maturity. Just growing older and realizing that my mother had an incurable illness, and that while I was growing up, she was truly doing the best that she could. I began to have compassion for her, even if we still weren't "close." I have wished in the past that I could go back in time and meet my mother as a teenager before she became ill—to see what she was like when she was "well"—to be her friend. I think she really must have needed a friend to talk to back then, but didn't have anyone who she could trust or anyone who could understand.*

How To Help a Sibling Deal With Your Disorder

Maybe it's not a parent who's having trouble dealing—maybe it's your brother or sister who doesn't understand what you're going through, resents all the attention you're getting, or wishes you would just deal with your problems on your own—whatever they are—and stop upsetting the family.

What can you do to reach out to your siblings? Maybe *he's* the one who can't deal with his emotions. Maybe *she's* in denial or can't understand why she's making your life a living

What Can I Do When My Parents Can't Deal?

When you know you need help but your parents refuse to acknowledge your problem, here are some things you can explain to help bridge the communication gap:

• Talk about your level of emotional distress in terms they can relate to and understand. Remember to consider your audience. Seek to communicate on their level.

• Discuss the link between your behavior and your emotions. You've tried other "quick fixes" and they have failed to work.

• Mental illness is a biological disease. You are not pretending to feel miserable. This is not something that will go away on its own.

• Make analogies to other diseases. Focus on the ones that you can't see but are potentially life-threatening if left untreated, such as diabetes and heart disease.

• Having a mental disorder does not mean that you are "crazy."

• Many famous people throughout history have had mental disorders and have been successfully treated.

• Mental disorders are treatable and can be improved within a relatively short time frame, the specifics of which will depend on your disorder.

• You are aware of the stigma associated with having a mental issue and are prepared to deal with it in order to take the necessary steps to recover; that stigma is hardly an issue compared to the level of pain you are suffering.

• Your mental disorder is not a reflection of their parenting. You do not see it as their fault. If anything, if you just had their support, you would feel safer and more able to focus on healing.

hell. If that is the situation, then take control. Try to educate your sibling about the disorder, the warning signs, what it's like for someone like you, who is suffering.

Your sibling may not know how to react to the truth of your disorder—or worse, may not even want to listen. Depending on how severe the situation is, you may have to deal with the fact that he or she *won't* talk to you. You may have to find another family member or a friend who can help you deal with your disappointment and your disorder. Just because your sibling has turned away from you does not necessarily mean that you'll have to let go of him or her forever. But if it does come to that, it will hurt. The pain can intensify any self-hate, insecurity, or anger that you may have, which is why you'll need to talk about it.

It's hard for people who have never been through a mental disorder to understand its severity. If your sibling seems resistant, try to understand his or her perspective. This person knew you for a long time, and then watched you change. This can cause confusion, anger, or doubt that you'll ever return to your former self. He or she may think you should just "get over it," or worse—may not even believe that you are ill. It may feel impossible to communicate the way you used to. You may have to alter your relationship and learn to live with it, at least for a while, if you can talk about everything but your disorder. Or you may only edit yourself during the holidays so that your sibling is less confrontational. Or, you may decide to disclose everything all at once, no matter the consequences.

As hurtful as your sibling's reaction may be, you cannot control him or her. The only person you can control is you. We can't tell you exactly what to do in every situation. But we can remind you that family can be extremely unique and complicated. This is true for everyone on the planet. Just remember that you are not alone in your struggle to meaningfully connect to the people you love. We're all working towards the same thing, in our own way. Chances are, your sibling wants the same thing you do. With a little patience and a lot of love, it's likely that you will eventually persevere.

The Flip Side

But maybe you're in the opposite situation. Maybe you're not the one looking for help and support from your family to deal with your disorder—maybe it's your family members who need help. *Then* what can you do?

If Your Parent is Suffering

We've all been embarrassed by our parents at some point. There's your mom standing in the parking lot after school waving and yelling your name. Your dad raps in front of your friends as he drives you to football practice. You feel totally helpless as a tidal wave of embarrassment washes over you. You think you may even drown. You may even flip out, declaring that you hate them. You sometimes wish they weren't there, or even worse, you wish they weren't your parents. You yell and scream. Eventually, you calm down. You realize they are going to be there for a long time, whether you like it or not. The other option—moving out, getting a job, and supporting yourself—isn't the best thing, either. So the next time they embarrass you, maybe you can try to remember that it isn't *that* bad.

Did You Know?

If someone in your family has a diagnosable mental disorder, you have a greater chance of developing it yourself. There is a biological link in families with mental disorders that shows they can be passed on much like cancer or heart problems. Environment can also play a role in the development of a mental disorder. The way you are raised will affect you for the rest of your life. The good news is that there are a lot of resources out there to help both you and your family. Many of them are listed for you at the end of this book.

But what if your parent has a mental disorder? What if you are the kid with the "psycho" parent who flips out, drinks too much, disappears for months at a time, or maybe even ends up in the hospital? How do you deal? When you are the kid people feel sorry for or the one who gets teased, you constantly live under a cloud of shame. You never know what to expect. Some days your home is quiet. Other times it's filled with anger. Or maybe your parent is too drunk or high most of the time to function normally. These experiences create painful memories that can last forever.

MARTHA's mother suffers from schizophrenia. *As a little girl, some kids on my block found out that my mom had schizophrenia and delusions. My sister and I had confided in one girl who lived on the block that our mother was saying that she was "Gizmo" from the movie Gremlins, and she then told her cousin, who also happened to be the neighborhood bully. So for a time, all of the boys on the block would shout 'MARTHA'S MOTHER THINKS SHE'S GIZMO! MARTHA'S MOTHER IS CRAZY!' whenever they saw me. It was mortifying, and was one of the first hard lessons I learned about trust.*

If you can relate to this, you're not alone. Pretty much every family in this country has at least one member with a mental disorder. Obviously some are more severe than others, but it's more universal than you probably imagine. If this is your situation, you may have a lot of unsettling questions. Am I going to end up like that person? What about my kids? What can I do to make sure I turn out "normal?"

What Can I Do When My Parent Has a Disorder?

- **Educate yourself on their disorder.** Learn the warning signs. Know the symptoms. The more you know about the disorder, the easier it will be to recognize it in yourself, should you begin to experience similar symptoms.

- **Ask questions.** Does anyone else in the family have this disorder? What other disorders might they have? Has anyone ever committed suicide? Education from books is one thing, but hearing personal stories and how people coped can be even more helpful in this situation.

- **Research treatment plans.** What plan is most effective for the disorder in question? For most disorders, research shows a combination of therapy and medication may work best. If you're concerned that your parent isn't getting the proper treatment, try reaching out to them or to another close family friend or relative to discuss options.

- **Talk about your feelings.** Discuss your thoughts and feelings about the disorder with someone you trust. Don't suppress your emotions. They will only come out sideways, which usually results in unhealthy behaviors. Take control of your feelings before they start to control you.

- **Be selective.** It isn't necessary that everyone know or understand that your parent has a mental disorder. After you educate yourself, you may see that this is a health issue, but unfortunately not everyone will agree with you. We would love to change everyone's view on mental disorders, but it will be better for you to be careful about who you tell. First make sure the people closest to you are on your team and care about you and your family.

- **Come to terms with your past.** Mental disorders can cause very specific family dynamics to take hold. They can change or reverse roles, so suddenly you're the parent (and your mom's acting like the child). Do everything you can to learn about families who have suffered from the disorder. Many people say that they will never repeat the same mistakes their parents made, but how will they know—or keep themselves from repeating the behavior—if they never understand what was behind them?

- **Be aware of yourself.** If you start experiencing the disorder on any level, seek help immediately. The earlier you get into treatment, the faster you can return to a sense of normalcy.

- **Embrace your individuality!** Just because someone in your family has a problem does not mean that you are fated to follow in those footsteps. With some disorders (like substance abuse), you have a choice. And the more you learn about the disorder, the better prepared you will be to chart your *own* future.

Bottom line: become a mini-expert on the disorder. This will help you for the rest of your life, whether or not you develop the illness. There is no guarantee that the education will prevent every major episode, but it will prepare you should you ever face the disorder—in yourself or someone you love.

If Your Sibling is Suffering

Sometimes it isn't a parent that experiences a disorder. When Ross was a child, it was his oldest brother. Ross grew up in a typical middle-class family in rural northeastern Pennsylvania, the youngest of three sons. His brother Vance is two-and-a-half years older, and his brother Thad is seven years older. Growing up, usually everything was great. They took regular family trips and did a lot together.

The typical childhood doesn't always stay that way, though. When Ross was in sixth grade he learned that Thad was in a psychiatric hospital.

Ross's family soon educated themselves on bipolar disorder. They took Thad to see a psychiatrist and psychologist and made sure he was taking his medications as prescribed. Eventually, Thad's disorder stabilized; he returned to PENN one year later and graduated with a degree in physics. Soon after, he began a doctoral program at Florida State University.

Thad's life finally looked like it was coming together again, but internally it was a different story.

ROSS *From the outside, everything appeared to be great, but it wasn't so good behind closed doors. Thad and my par-*

ents fought endlessly. He would go weeks without speaking to them, and when they would finally talk it would always result in a heated argument. Eventually, Thad told my parents that he never wanted to speak to them again. He cut off all communication and moved to Florida. I was 16 at the time. I felt like I had lost my best friend and didn't know whether to turn my anger towards my brother or my parents.

Ross's struggle is fairly universal. Have you been there? Have you ever watched a sibling become highly emotional for no obvious reason? Why does he cry so much? Why did she hit you? Why can't he get along with Mom and Dad for just one night so you can sleep? Why can't she snap out of it, whatever it is?

When you educate yourself on your sibling's disorder, you can begin to find out the answers to some of these questions. You open a door to better communication and potentially to a healthier relationship. By learning more, you can ask specific questions about the disorder, which could get the conversation rolling. But even if the conversation doesn't go anywhere, you'll gain insight into how the disorder affects your sibling. This will make it easier to have patience as he or she starts to heal. And don't forget; healthy communication is a process. It won't happen overnight. It could take time for your sibling to find the right words to express herself, and more importantly, to feel comfortable talking to you about deep, emotional issues. Maybe your sister feels like she's failed you or the family. Or she could be angry. She could be riding a wave of many differing and confusing emotions. The best thing you can do is to share your willingness to talk, and to be there whenever she needs you.

Maybe you have a great relationship with your brother or sister and you can talk about anything. In this situation, dealing with a mental disorder can deepen your relationship, while also helping to make you more sensitive and caring. Your sibling will probably sense your level of care and your interest in how they are healing. This could help them feel safe turning to you whenever they are scared or vulnerable.

If your sibling doesn't *want* to seek help, there is very little that you can do for them. You may have to watch him hit rock bottom. Regardless, you will need to be particularly vigilant about taking care of your own mental health along the way. Talk to someone you trust about your reactions—your feelings, hopes, disappointment, pain—so that you can maintain *your* sense of self as your sibling struggles to find their way.

ALISON's brother took his own life when she was in her first year of college. *On that Friday, March 24, I spent much of the day outside studying, as it was a beautiful, sunny day in Philadelphia. When I returned to my dorm room at about 5 p.m., I turned on my computer. The phone in our dorm room rang, and in typical fashion, I didn't answer it. Three minutes later, it rang again. Five minutes after that, it rang once more.*

After the third time, I dialed in to my voice mail messages to see if any of the calls were for me. The first message I heard was from my grandmother, who lived just an hour from my campus. She said "Ali, it's okay, we'll be there soon." Totally confused, I listened to my next message. It was from my mom, and in a shaky voice she said "Ali, it's Mommy. Call me at home." She never referred to herself as "Mommy."

I hung up and called home, and a strange voice answered. The woman immediately recognized my voice and said, "Alison, it's Jo. Let me put your mom on the phone." I had no idea what was happening. My mom came on the line and said, "Ali...Brian shot himself." I collapsed on the cold wooden floor. "Is he okay?" I asked, thinking they must be on their way to the hospital. But she replied, "No, honey...he's dead."

A few hours, and a long, silent car ride with my grandparents later, I was home. I walked inside and immediately saw my father, who hadn't been to our house for over 10 years. He didn't belong there; this whole scene was surreal. My mom then emerged out of the throngs of people who were gathered around. She wrapped her arms around me and we sobbed together.

By around 10 p.m., most everyone had left, and my mom and I sat together at our kitchen table. We discussed the plans for the weekend. She told me that she, my stepfather and my father would be going to the funeral home in the morning to pick out a casket. They would then go to the cemetery to pick out a gravesite, and then our rabbi would be coming over that evening to talk to us all about Brian, so he could proceed over his funeral the next day. I told her I wanted to go, too. I didn't want the last decisions about Brian to be made without me.

The conversation wound down. All I could say was, "Part of me just doesn't believe he's dead, but at the same time, part of me almost feels like he died a year-and-a-half ago." It had been a year-and-a-half since Brian had sought help for the mental health issues he had been experiencing in college. But it had also been that long since my normally outgoing, funny, gregarious big brother had been any of those things. He suffered in silence for years without asking for help. And by the time he did seek help, Brian had already lost so much of himself. Sadly, it just took another year-and-a-half for us to ultimately lose him, too.

When Alison returned to campus, she searched endlessly for resources to help her process her grief over losing her brother. She figured that if this could happen to Brian, then it could happen to anyone. She found comfort in the realization that

Did You Know?

Suicide is the second leading cause of death on college campuses. In 2004, over 32,000 Americans took their own lives—a large percentage of whom had no real desire to actually die. They just didn't feel they could go on living, feeling the way they did. This is why *seeking help* is so important—it doesn't have to be that way.

she wasn't alone. But in a way, she was. At the time, Alison discovered there were no campus groups promoting mental health or offering resources for suicide prevention. This inspired her to take action and start **Active Minds**, a peer-to-peer outreach group founded to help educate students about mental health issues. After Alison graduated she set out to expand the organization nationwide, and today there are nearly 100 **Active Minds** chapters across the United States.

Family *Matters*

A family will be more successful in dealing with any mental disorder when most—or all—of the following things are true: the disorder is recognized early, the person affected is willing to seek help and comply with the treatment plan, and the family plays an active role in the person's recovery. There are endless success stories of families where this has been the case.

Some families are more fortunate than others. They may recognize a disorder early on, when a child is in lower or middle school. They may have insurance or find a way to easily afford treatment. They may be able to work well as a team to develop positive coping mechanisms.

Sometimes the child needs an extended break from school to successfully deal with the problem. Or the parents may need to work with the school in order to devise an ongoing plan. Regardless, learning the lifestyle changes and coping mechanisms necessary to successfully navigate a disorder will be critical, especially as a child grows older. The brain will continue to develop, and this will enable the child to handle the issue with more maturity, and possibly less supervision.

Families That Eat Together...Stay Together

Young people whose families regularly eat dinner together are less likely to be depressed or use drugs than those whose families don't. They are also less likely to be violent, engage in sexual activity, and experience emotional stress. Regularly shared mealtimes can increase a sense of belonging, stability, and the entire family's feeling of group connection.

The dinner example above was included to remind you of the importance of *community*. Eating dinner as a family is helpful because it creates a connection at home, so you aren't as inclined to run out and try to find that connection somewhere else instead—like in a bottle, a drug, or a bad relationship. If you had this connection growing up, it may serve to help you now. But if you didn't, then you may need to work on creating a community outside of your home. That can be done in a number of ways, like through team sports, a fraternity or sorority, or even just having a solid group of close friends.

Many of the effects of family relationships stay with us for a lifetime. You can learn a lot by tracing your past, so don't be afraid to start. If you aren't happy with the state of things in your family, remember Martha's story. There can be hope in even the darkest of situations, but it may not come easy. If there is one thing guaranteed about family, it's that there will always be some hard times. Hopefully you'll be able to work through them together, and in doing so, manage to find a deeper understanding of yourself *and* the people you love.

CHAPTER 6

BEYOND YOUR BUDDY LIST:
Real Friendships

"And I would have
stayed up with you all night,
Had I known how to save a life."
—**The Fray "How to Save a Life"**

ROSS *My best friends are the ones who have been with me ever since I first started experiencing the mood swings, the violence, and the voices. They have sat next to me as I crouched in fear from hallucinations of a man chasing me or sitting behind me. They have watched helplessly as I punched things or put* *my fists through walls. In the beginning, none of them really knew what to do or say to me. One of my friends said once that he just thought I was having a "bad day," or that whatever I was going through would pass. They had no awareness of these things, so what could they do? On a lot of levels they could only do so much, because I wasn't really receptive to the idea of getting help anyway.*

My friendships continued this way for at least four years. My friends would be there to listen every time I broke down. They were there to pick me up when I passed out, and help me to at least get inside the house. They would clean up my parties while I was puking. They really wanted to help me to feel better, but didn't know exactly what I needed until I could find a way to tell them, and—most importantly—until I was willing to accept their help.

These friends saw a huge change in me after I hit rock bottom. (They originally thought my "rock bottom" was back in high school when I was first hospitalized for wanting to take my own life, but the reality is that I was even closer to death in the years to follow.) Probably the biggest change they noticed was that I was now more willing to try to figure out productive ways to deal with my disorder. I gradually started to tell my friends whenever I wasn't comfortable doing something, and they would respond by trying to not put me in that situation. I would also let my friends know when they would do or say something that bothered me, and they would try their best to help by no longer saying or doing those things.

After my close friends were able to adjust to some things for me, I started to have a thicker skin if they would ever crack a joke about me, or my problems. Nothing mean, but just the way that friends joke around with each other. I was able to loosen up a lot, because I knew they cared and weren't trying to hurt me. It took a while for me to get to that point, but I didn't want everyone walking on eggshells or always focused on me when something went wrong. Part of this process was learning enough about my disorder so that I could verbalize what it was that I needed.

At one point, I was engaged to be married, but it didn't work out, and the relationship ended. After the breakup, my friends were there for me every single day. My phone rang constantly. People made efforts to visit and spend time with me. We learned a lot about one another during that time. They knew that such a devastating change in my life could kill me, because they had been through so much with me for so long, and we had even talked about it. Some friends would call to talk and ask questions, while others would just sit and listen. The changes in all of them—over those seven years since we had left high school—meant more to me than anything in the world.

But I also think my friends would be the first ones to tell you that I also do a ton of things for them, and that the relationship is mutual. They never gave up on me, but I never gave up on them either. I plan things, and usually tend to be seen as the "responsible" one in the group. Because I travel so much, I'm fortunate enough to able to keep in close touch with everyone and keep them all up to date. Part of my maintenance is to talk to my friends constantly. I wouldn't know any other way to live! The father of one of my friends told me that he appreciates how much we have all been able to stay together through the years. This disorder, while terrifying, challenging, and difficult, *has helped me to become more sensitive to other people's feel-ings and needs. So if my friends ever need anything, they know they can call—and I'll be there—no matter what. It's funny, because I was their measuring bar of sanity for so long. But now the focus is not so much on me anymore, as it is on who-ever in the group might need to talk, and when. I know that my friends are very proud of me, and I am just as proud of them.*

Friendships and Mental Health

There are all kinds of friendships in life. Some are based on convenience, and others on true compatibility. Most people have few "real" friends. And even some of those real friends will feel stumped when dealing with problems, par-ticularly those related to mental health. That's not to say that these friends don't care. But friendships can become chal-lenging or strained when dealing with a mental disorder.

Mental disorders can change the dynamics of friendships. Many people want to know what role a friend should play when dealing with serious personal issues. Some of us aren't even sure we have the time to help our friends. We're too busy balancing everything going on in our own lives. Others *want* to help, but they don't even know where to begin, let alone *what* to say or *who* to go to for answers.

And we're not always sure how much responsibility we should take on. How much can—or should—you help some-one who is suffering? Will your friend appreciate the help? And will you feel good about it, or will you start to feel bur-dened and resentful, as if it's your *job* to make your friend feel better? If you do want to help them, but you don't know where to start, then this chapter can offer some help. And if *you* are the person suffering from a disorder and have no idea how to handle your friends, this chapter is a good one for you, too.

Pain Knows Pain: Destructive Friendships

Maybe some of this sounds familiar: You're desperate to find someone who gets you, who understands your pain. Someone who knows what it's like to live on the dark side. To smash knuckles into walls. Spend endless nights without sleep. Starve. Feel the razor blade cut into your flesh. It's a relief to find such a person because you have so much in common. You suddenly feel validated when your deepest secrets are understood.

Emotions are contagious: *pain attracts pain.* In some ways, it's comforting when the people around you mirror your own internal state, especially when you're suffering. The cliché "misery loves company" could not be more true. But if you really want to help yourself, one of the best conscious decisions you can make is to surround yourself with people who *aren't* totally invested in living on the dark side.

It's easy to bond with someone who not only understands your pain, but feeds it. The problem with this type of friendship is that you connect with someone who is equally focused on his problem. He either runs from it or dwells on it, and that's the main thing you have in common. Together, you try doing things that deepen your feelings, whatever they may be. And it can be thrilling to find someone who "gets it," who likes getting messed up as much as you. Hey—he may even teach you some new tricks.

This is a common type of "friendship," and one that rarely ends well. You will often see it in young women with eating disorders, as they tend to seek out others with the same problem. The disorder becomes almost like a competition. They binge. They purge. They compete to see who can eat the least, lose the most weight, or hate their bodies most fiercely. There are also young men with various disorders who find a release in fighting or drinking together. They act out in different ways, but the person with the most anger always wins.

In chapter two we talked about Tyrone, who grew up in a family that was deeply entrenched in the gang culture. His father was in a gang, and so were his brothers. They beat him from the time he was three, until he got big enough to fight back. Violence was the language they used to express themselves and to bond with one another. The only way Tyrone was taught to express emotions was through violence. It was all he knew, so it was nearly impossible to break the pattern. Ross first met Tyrone when he was in juvenile hall, just as he was coming to terms with how his childhood had turned him into the person he had become.

Tyrone was taught to hate the world and to express that feeling through violence. He made "friends" with people who spoke the same language. They acted out together, seeking out fights to express their rage. They had no other way to release it. Tyrone's "friends" would high-five him when he broke eye sockets or skulls, but he couldn't find any of them when he wanted to change. No one came to visit him in juvenile hall. No one was there when the police showed up. Suddenly, he found himself alone.

Tyrone is obviously an extreme case, but the truth still holds: you bond with what you know. It's very common to fall into "friendships" with people who feel familiar to you, who may (and not necessarily even on purpose) make it easier for you to continue old patterns of behavior. It may feel good and it may be all you know, but there *is* a way out. Breaking the pattern of these friendships can be painful and difficult. In doing so, you're asking yourself to go against everything you may have learned. The old, destructive behavior could feel like home. But you're not fated to live there forever. There *are* things you can do. It takes a lot of work to develop new connections with healthier, more positive people—but it is possible, and well worth the effort.

Finding Others Like You

Just as people connect in the midst of a dysfunction, it's also possible to bond in health. There *are* people who are dedicated to overcoming their problems. They know what it's like to go through pain, but can also see past it. They want a life. They are determined to change for the better.

If you meet such a person who is in recovery or treatment, you need to make sure that he or she is dedicated to getting healthy, rather than dwelling on old problems. You can actively seek out people who share your issues. Many pursue Twelve Step programs to find like-minded people in recovery. Alcoholics Anonymous has *sponsors*, people who have been in the program for a while who want to help others with their recovery. Sponsors guide *sponsees*, people who are new to the program or who may need extra help in getting well. This arrangement can work well, because the sponsor has already experienced the sponsee's pain.

You can meet other people who share your issues almost anywhere, if you're open to it. Think about it. When 20 to 25%

of people out there have a mental disorder, your chances of meeting someone who shares or understands your problem are quite significant. You are not alone. But it's not enough for a new friend just to share your problem. The person also needs to have a desire to *do something about it.*

BOB was diagnosed with anxiety disorder. *I always liked seeing my friends, but never really felt that anyone understood all of me—or my anxiety–until I met someone who had the same problem. Meeting him was really freeing for me. It was like we instantly knew each other, like he knew what it was like to be me. We soon turned our instant connection into a solid friendship, one that has given us both an opportunity to learn better ways of coping with anxiety and grow into more stable people.*

Friendships that form under these circumstances can be more "real" than any you've ever had before. A friend like this can be there when others have failed you. He can help you when you feel like giving up. She can remind you that you're not alone, that you're not the only one out there with these problems. The ways that these "real" friends can help you are nearly endless, and the bonds can last for a lifetime. You have a stronger foundation and an understanding of one another that is rooted in something much deeper than pain. Friends like this can sometimes mean more to you than many previous relationships because they are all about support, and how you can help each other to live a better life.

COLLEEN suffers from anxiety, depression, anorexia and bulimia. *My friends are immensely supportive in all areas of my life, especially where my emotional health is concerned. When I was in ninth grade I was pulled out of boarding school and put into a mental hospital. When I got out, I started to attend public high school. I was a new student in the middle of the spring semester, so naturally everyone wondered where I had come from. I made a conscious choice to be honest about what I had been through, and I have never regretted it. It turns out that many of the people I met either knew people with mental health issues or they had them, too. So as a result, I now have a handful of amazing women in my life.*

My friend Chandler never allows me to wallow or apologize for myself. I can recall a card she wrote me in my senior year of college that said, "We will get through this"—because she said "we," not just "you." My friend Lindsay is a nurse now. She is probably the most supportive friend I have in terms of my eating disorder. She has the healthiest self-image of any woman I know, but she totally gets it.

Lindsay listens to me whenever I am irrationally hysterical about having eaten something fattening or if I've gained a few pounds. She always brings me back to reality. She empa-

thizes with me, but also helps me to gain perspective—she reminds me that it's not the end of the world to gain and lose a little weight, or to eat some chocolate once in a while. She compliments me when my weight is healthy and celebrates the little victories along with me.

My friends Tera and Annie are both dealing with mental health issues of their own. So when they support me, they do it just by simply being there, by understanding. We don't always need words between us to know what the other person is going through, as we've all been there.

Telling Your Friends About Your Problems: Will They Understand?

Telling a friend that you have a mental disorder can be a hard thing on many levels. It can bring up many of your insecurities and vulnerabilities. Will this person understand you? Judge you? Make fun of you? Even worse, will your friend abandon you? We depend on our friends for so many things. It may seem easier to stay silent rather than risk losing the relationship. But then, aren't you living a lie? We can't expose the depth of our souls to everyone, as that's just not realistic. But you need to be able to tell your close friends about your emotions. Your feelings are a major part of who you are, especially if you have a mental disorder.

Finding the right words can be equally challenging. Something traumatic can happen so quickly, and at first you may not know what to say, or who you can trust.

ALISON lost her brother to suicide. *For me, it was extremely difficult to reach out to my friends afterward. They were incredibly supportive; many even came home from college and others sent cards or left encouraging phone messages, but I didn't totally know how to share what all I was feeling with them. I remember also thinking that I would never wish this pain on anyone, so I hesitated sharing the depth of my suffering pain as I didn't want them to have to feel it, too. For about six months, I just tried to keep it inside.*

Slowly, I learned how to grieve more openly. My friends became my grieving board: friends from both home and college allowed me to open up and finally start taking care of myself, as opposed to my always worrying about everyone else. They have continued to be the most openhearted, enlightened, understanding group of people I have ever met. They admitted that they couldn't know exactly what I was going through, but they let me talk and wanted to listen to what I had to say.

It's normal to fear your friends' judgments. It's also normal to expect them to judge you. But very often, that fear isn't even real. It's imagined. In some ways it can be easier to think this way—to stay silent—no one could ever possibly get you, so why even try? But if you act this way, you're not even giving your friends the chance to support you. Maybe they *won't* judge you. Maybe they'll be like Alison's friends, and help you to make peace with some of your issues. The point is, you'll never know unless you try, and having the support of a close friend can make all the difference.

It probably feels safer on some level to be miserable and lonely—than to risk sharing your emotions and possibly feeling like an idiot. But here's the deal: *everyone* has problems. Maybe not all as dire as yours, but if you continue to live in your own bubble, you'll never really know.

Alison became closer to her friends and they developed deeper bonds when she was finally able to share her feelings with them. Like Alison, you need to give your friends a chance, and see what kind of people they really are.

It can be very disappointing when your friends don't understand you. But even then, there's still hope.

MARTHA was diagnosed with depression. One of her friends had a hard time understanding what she was going through. *Shirley and I stopped talking as often as we used to, because I started to feel like I had to take care of her feelings, and I'm guessing that she felt at a loss as to how to relate to me in my depressive state.*

I was uncomfortable with the lack of understanding and felt I should reach out to her. I told Shirley that I was taking an antidepressant to help with my depression. Shirley told me she didn't believe depression was a real problem, that I should be able to just "snap out of it" if I really wanted to. I was devastated. I know it's hard for people who haven't experienced the severity of a mental disorder to understand its emotional complexity. But I also felt that Shirley's comment had nothing to do with me so much as it was a reflection of her own belief system.

I told her that I was not making a choice to be depressed, and that if I could, I certainly would not be choosing to feel so terrible all the time. Why wouldn't I want to feel good? I asked her to consider my mother who is diagnosed with paranoid schizophrenia, has suffered from depression, and has been on medication most of her adult life. Is my mom just "choosing" to feel bad?

At first, Shirley was silent. She finally said, "You know, half the time I don't know exactly what to say to you about this stuff."

It was in that moment that I realized it was Shirley's limitations about what to do that made our friendship awkward. My getting angry with her wouldn't change a thing. I explained to Shirley that she didn't have to know what to say to me about depression; that all I needed was for her to listen attentively and offer some compassion. Shirley told me she would try—and thankfully, we are still friends to this day.

Not everyone is going to possess the skills needed to deal with the extreme states of these disorders. But very often, we just need someone to *listen*. We need to know that someone cares about us and supports us. Our true friends can do this. And this is another reason to learn as much as you can about your disorder: so you can better explain it to those people who are closest to you.

CLARENCE came to better understand what a friend with bipolar disorder was going through. *I had never personally experienced depression or any other mental disorder, so when my friend first started going through a lot of changes, I really just thought he wanted attention or that he was just making it up. It took me a while to realize that someone would have to want attention really badly to make up the sorts of things he was saying and doing—that there had to be something a lot more serious going on. That's when I started to really believe that he had bipolar disorder.*

You may wish that your friend could take away your pain. So when they can't fix you, it's common to think, "*No one knows what to do for me.*" This can make you feel empty, even hopeless. But remember, no one can read your mind. It's impossible for them to know how they can help you, unless you *tell them.* The more educated and confident you become, the better you will be able to handle situations with friends who may genuinely want to help you, but just don't know how.

What Happens When Your Friend Leaves You?

Most of us have probably lost a friend at some point, for one reason or another. Perhaps the person hurt you somehow, or maybe you went through some changes—and they didn't change with you. No matter what the scenario is, it *sucks*. Plain and simple. It can really hurt. You get so used to seeing her smile, or joking around with him every day, or having meaningful conversations, or just the general routine of hanging out together, so that when it's suddenly gone, you really miss it.

Unfortunately, losing a friend can be far too common when you are experiencing a mental disorder. Most people don't know much about mental disorders, and some aren't willing to learn. In some cases, the person simply isn't capable of dealing with your issue. Maybe it's too close to home. Maybe this friend has issues of his own that he's not prepared to face, and so seeing you dealing with your issues scares him. There are endless reasons why someone may stop being your friend, but whatever the reason, nothing hurts more than being abandoned. Some friends will let you know exactly what the problem is or why they are leaving, and others will just disappear. You may wonder if they left because they decided they don't like you, or because you did something to offend them. Are they ashamed of you because you tried to kill yourself? Do they understand that you don't want to feel so miserable all the time? Do they know how much you need them right now?

You can never really replace a lost friend. You can make new ones, and they will hopefully be even better, but you'll still have to mourn the loss. Eventually you'll move on with your life, make more friends, and find new things to do. But such a loss can bring real feelings of uncertainty, fear, anxiety, and anger to the surface. It's a lot to manage at once.

If a friend dumps you, you're also likely to feel more insecure about your disorder. There will be more anger and more self-hate directed toward this monster that you can't control. You may even feel like you can never trust anyone again, or that there's no end to what the disorder does to you. These feelings are totally legitimate, but you have to try to keep things in perspective and move forward with your life.

Your ex-friend does *not* represent everyone in the world. There are other people who *will* care about you. But you'll never find them if you don't learn from this experience (and when you do find them, you'll appreciate them that much more). You can start by working on all of the components we mentioned in chapter four. Learn everything you can about your disorder. The next time you develop a new friendship, you can let the person know what happened to you in the past. In time, you'll develop more courage to be honest about yourself, knowing that some people will have an easier time accepting you than others. And in the process, you'll find out who your true friends really are. You *can*, and you *WILL* get through this.

Communication Is Key

No matter how close you are to your friends, they can't possibly know every single thing you're thinking. Even the most intuitive friends will still need you to communicate with them. It may feel uncomfortable to put yourself out there at first, but it's unlikely that your needs will be met if you remain quiet and detached. This is the case with anyone, but it's all the more true if you suffer from a mental disorder.

Life actually simplifies when you communicate. It gives the people around you a chance to show up, or to move on. The "games" start to vanish. You begin to see people for who they are—the ones who can be there for you, the others that may try but still don't always seem to "get it," and the ones who will *never* really get it. Some of these realizations can hurt. You may discover that someone who you once loved and trusted cannot give you what you need. Or you could develop an even deeper bond with someone else who surprises you with compassion and understanding.

Witnessing destructive behavior can be devastating, not to mention totally confusing. Your friends may know that you're in trouble and need help, but sometimes they don't know how to make a difference. And when you don't share your needs, you and your friend can end up totally perplexed—and paralyzed. This is where many relationships unravel. How many times have you walked out on love or on a friendship because it got too scary? Because you felt too vulnerable? This is why communication is so important.

We're not talking about communication like, "I think I'll have the pasta for lunch." We're talking more along the lines of "Hey, I'm feeling nervous about sharing what's going on with me and I just need you to listen." Or "I love you, but I just need a little space right now." Give your friends the benefit of the doubt and try really talking to them about things. If they love you, they will want to give you what you need. But they'll never have the chance if you shut them out and only talk about things like pasta.

These kinds of friendships are not only possible, but they happen every day. There are good people who know how to handle being there for you. If you are in an unhealthy friendship, you can try to talk about it and give it some time. If the friend just doesn't get it, then focus on finding someone who does—someone who cares and who will be there for support. But also remember that in a healthy friendship, it can't be all about you. You also need to be there for your friends and be willing to help them, because most people will eventually give up on one-sided friendships.

If Your Friend Has A Mental Disorder

Maybe you're not the one who has the mental disorder. Perhaps you're getting worried about a friend. You've started to see some major changes in this person. You want to help. You do anything you think will help to bridge her back to health. You try to reach out. You tell her you're there for her, you care about her, and that she can talk to you about anything—that you won't judge her or disown her. But yet, she still ends up being hospitalized.

Or maybe you make a new friend who tells you he has a mental disorder. You feel like you want to be supportive, but you have no idea how you're supposed to react.

What can you do in these types of situations? Are you really as helpless as you feel? What can you say—or *should* you say? Much like we discussed in chapter four, the answer may be complex. There is no foolproof way to deal with a friend's mental disorder. Finding a mental health professional who may be able to help you understand what's going on is one of the best things you can do. Also, check out the "Resources" section in the back of this book to find out how you can learn more about your friend's condition, what you can do to help him or her, and what resources are available to offer YOU some help as well. There is a lot of information out there!

As we have said many times, these disorders affect everyone differently. There are many levels of severity. Treatment plans are rarely, if ever, the same. But let's say you're relatively inexperienced when it comes to dealing with mental disorders, and all you know about them is what you've seen on television. You don't know how to relate to your friend, but you desperately want to understand. If this is you, there are many things you can do.

Watch for the Signs

A campus outreach website (**www.halfofus.com**) for mental health issues, sponsored by *The Jed Foundation* and *mtvU*, offers the following warning signs as an indication that your friend may be dealing with more than just everyday stress:

- Feelings of hopelessness or being trapped
- Anxiety and agitation
- Impulsive, reckless behavior
- Social withdrawal
- Uncontrollable anger or feelings of revenge
- Fatigue
- Increased alcohol or drug use
- Inability to concentrate
- No appetite (or increased appetite)
- Dramatic mood swings
- Sense that life has no purpose
- No interest in activities
- Insomnia or increased sleeping
- Feelings of worthlessness or guilt
- Depressed mood
- Thoughts of death or suicide

You can better educate yourself about your friend's disorder by reading books and searching online. Just try any search engine, plug in the name of your friend's issue as your "search" term, and you'll find that the web has thousands of pages relating to mental disorders! You can also learn a lot about the *symptoms, warning signs, triggers, side effects* and *treatment plans* for each disorder by simply adding these words to your online search.

Once you feel adequately educated, it may be easier to approach your friend. But that doesn't mean that your friend will be ready to discuss the disorder. You must be respectful of his time and space. You can definitely say things like "*I care and want to be here for you.*" You can talk about the things you've learned, but your friend's experience may not be quite in line with all that you've read about, as disorders affect everybody differently. Be careful not to project the specifics of what you read onto your friend. It's better to just express empathy than to approach the conversation as if you already know everything. Otherwise, your friend is likely to shut down. And wouldn't you? No one wants to be told *how* they're feeling.

At first, it might be difficult for your friend to open up to you. Be prepared for this, and don't take it personally, as it may take a little time. If you want to hold onto the friendship, you'll need to be patient. Your friend might feel self-conscious, ashamed, afraid, inadequate—or all kinds of conflicting emotions, none of which has anything to do with you, or how this person feels about you. If she wants space, give it freely without any strings attached. Don't make her feel like she *owes* you an explanation or dissertation on what she's going through. Just let her know that the door is always open, and you will always be there.

When Your Friend is Released from the Psych Ward

It isn't always easy to know what to say or do once your friend is released from the psych ward. But why is that? If your friend got out of the hospital after breaking his leg, you would want to know how it happened, how it felt, how long he'll be in a cast, and if there is anything you can do for him. It's similar in the case of a mental disorder. You can ask your friend what happened, how it feels, what the treatment is like, and if there is anything you can do. Sometimes friends can be there to just listen. Let your friend vent if she wants to, and get it all out. It can be important to help her resume her normal routine, so she'll see she isn't confined by the disorder. But again, this will all depend on the individual. In the meantime, educating yourself, listening, and being supportive are all good places to start.

When Your Friend Shuts You Out

Oftentimes a friend may not be open to your offers to help them. Maybe he doesn't return phone calls. He doesn't hang out anymore. Or when you do see him, you seem to have nothing to talk about, as though he has nothing to say. Or maybe he still manages to maintain a social façade—the one he's always had—but you see straight through it.

Regardless of how your friend may have changed, one thing is clear to you: your friend is not doing well, and it seems there is nothing you can do. Every time you approach her, she shuts down and tells you, "I'm fine," "leave me alone," or "I don't have any problems." When she refuses your attempts to connect, it leaves you feeling hopeless and frustrated.

Ross frequently hears about these kinds of friendships. Here are some of the types of questions he hears most often after one of his presentations:

- My friend is constantly passing out from alcohol and drugs. He won't talk about it and refuses to stop using. *What can I do?*

- My friend hardly eats anymore. When she does eat, she goes into the bathroom right away. She looks awful and she won't listen to us. I'm scared for her. *What can I do?*

- My friend talks about suicide and death all the time. He cuts himself, breaks his knuckles on walls, and calls me at 2 a.m., telling me he wants to die. *What can I do?*

- My friend has just completely stopped doing everything that we used to do. I hardly see him anymore, and he just seems so out of it. *What can I do?*

- I have a friend who goes to another school. She texts me to tell me that she can't deal with anything anymore. She was diagnosed with a disorder in high school, but I know she isn't taking care of herself. *What can I do?*

"What can I do? What can I possibly do?" It's good to see so much concern for our friends out there, but there are just no easy answers. Each person's problem is unique to them. The best thing you can do is to sit down with a mental health

professional to try to learn more about your friend's disorder, and talk about how you see it affecting him or her. But here are some other things you can keep in mind.

How Can I Help My Friend?

- **Turn confrontation into conversation.** When you approach a friend about mental health issues, it can quickly turn into a confrontation. You're almost sure to hear, "I'm fine. You don't get it. Leave me alone." Here's what you have to focus on in these situations—just take a deep breath and think about how *to turn the confrontation...into a conversation.*

- **Help your friend feel comfortable.** Your friend may be defensive because he thinks you're judging him. You can quickly change this by reminding him you're on the same team. You care about him. You're not there to argue; you're there to help. You miss him, and you want to be there for him. Offer to go to with him to therapy. He may decline, but it might help him feel more comfortable just to know that you cared enough to offer.

- **Discuss the reasons.** Refer back to chapter two, where we discussed the most common reasons why people don't seek help. Reread the chapter with your friend in mind. Does your friend feel weak? Stupid? Afraid you will call her crazy? These are some of the questions to consider when you want to start a conversation.

- **Approach you friend in a familiar way.** Think about how you used to enjoy spending time together. Did you watch TV? Shoot hoops? Sometimes people say they want to approach a friend about his problems, so they decide to take him for a walk. But here's the thing—if you've never taken a walk with your friend before, then this is not the time to start. Think about it. You're doing something with

(more)

How Can I Help My Friend? (cont.)

them that you've never done, while you're looking to discuss the person's deepest, darkest issues. This situation will feel anything but natural to them, and will likely *not* put them at ease.

If you're worried about a friend you have known for a long time, then simply doing something you used to do together is a good option. Maybe you always went for coffee, to the gym, or did something healthy together to relieve your stress. One of these situations would provide a good setting for you to have the conversation.

- **Talk face-to-face.** For most people today, interactivity is like oxygen. Instant messaging is an essential part of life. It's a fast, easy way to communicate. You can talk about anything—even the tough stuff. It's essentially "non-confrontational confrontation." Meaning, you can argue with someone over IM...while they sit 10 feet away from you in the same room! It's often more comfortable than actually talking to the person face-to-face, especially if you're mad. Avoidance only takes a "click."

  But if you are using instant messaging or texting in order to address emotional problems with your friend, she can just choose not to reply. If you post on her profile, she doesn't have to publish it. You can play these games forever. Where will it get you? Be the bigger person. Talk to your friend—face-to-face. You'll have a much better chance of resolving your issues—or getting her to open up.

- **You can't be a therapist or psychologist.** What you absolutely cannot do, no matter how much you love your friend, is stand in for a therapist or psychologist. You can't diagnose your friend's problems, recommend treatment, or prescribe him medication. And this is the reality, no matter how much you think you may know about his disorder. It's natural to want to heal him, but the best way to help your friend is simply to support and empower him as he comes to terms with his illness and tries to resume his life.

- **You cannot help someone unless the person wants help.** Regardless of the severity of your friend's disorder, if she doesn't *want* help there is nothing you can do. Trust us on this. You can still follow many of the suggestions outlined in this book and try to open the door, but you cannot control the outcome. You cannot control how your friend will respond to your attempts to help her. This should not stop you from trying; it's just a lesson in life. Remember that you cannot control anyone...but yourself.

- **Take care of yourself, too!** When dealing with a friend who has a mental disorder, or anytime you're trying to navigate a difficult situation, you also have to take responsibility for your *own* health. If your friend is locked in a downward spiral, don't forget to do what you need to do in order to protect yourself. Talk to someone you trust and get the support you need. Otherwise, these problems can suck you into the undertow before you know it. It's important to want to be supportive of your friends, but don't neglect your own health in the process—take care of yourself first.

- **Remember that caring about your friend can't make your friend care about herself.** This may sound crazy, but bear with us. When someone has a lot of self-hate, it's almost impossible for him to receive love. You may tell him you love him, but it just doesn't register. It can't. He, like many others who feel this way, sees no reason why you *would* love him. Until he can learn to love himself, he is only able to see his flaws and faults. This should not keep you from expressing your affection, but just realize what you're up against. And don't lose your faith in him. Maybe you can eventually help him to see himself through your eyes. And of course, encourage him to seek professional help as well.

Sometimes it's too painful to stay in a friendship with someone who doesn't see a way out, and continues to destroy himself. If he was a friend who helped *you* get out of a destructive situation and then slipped back into his problems, you may feel compelled to stay. You care about this friend on every level imaginable, and it hurts to see him this way. But if it gets to the point where the friendship is toxic and no longer healthy for you, then you may need to distance yourself. At this point, you will have tried everything you can, but the nature of the friendship will have changed so much that it no longer resembles the friendship as *you* remember it. It can be an extremely painful decision to have to make, but you may need to ultimately end the friendship. If it comes to this, let him know why—you may even tell him that the door is always open, should he choose to rekindle your friendship.

How Can I Help a Friend Who's Suicidal?

The Jed Foundation offers this advice (adapted from the American Association of Suicidology) when dealing with a suicidal friend:

- Don't try to manage the situation alone. It is often best to include others when helping someone who is at risk for suicide.

- Be aware—learn the risk factors and warning signs for suicide and where you can get help.

- Be direct—talk openly and matter-of-factly about suicide, what you have observed, and what your concerns are regarding his/her well-being.

- Be willing to listen—allow the expression of feelings, accept those feelings, and be patient.

- Be non-judgmental—don't debate whether suicide is right or wrong, or whether the person's feelings are good or bad. Don't give a lecture on the value of life.

- Be available—show interest, understanding, and support.

- Don't dare him/her to do it.

- Don't act shocked.

- Don't ask "why."

- Don't agree to be "sworn to secrecy."

- Offer hope that alternatives are available—but don't offer reassurances that any one alternative will turn things around.

- Take action—remove lethal means of self-harm such as pills, ropes, and alcohol or other drugs.

- Get help from others with more experience and expertise.

- Be actively involved in encouraging the person to see a mental health professional.

- **Don't leave the person alone** until help is available.

Individuals contemplating suicide often don't believe that they *can* be helped, so you may have to be active and persistent in helping them to get the help they need. In addition, after helping a friend during a mental health crisis, be aware of how *you* may have been affected emotionally and seek the necessary support for yourself.

If Your Friend Talks About Suicide

If your friend talks about suicide or taking his own life, it can be frightening, and really hard to know what you should do. You may think he's just doing it to get attention or sympathy. But most likely, it's a call for help. In that moment, there's no way to know how serious your friend is, but why flirt with disaster? Why take that chance? *Ask your friend if he has a specific plan in mind.* If he does, try to get help for him *immediately.* You may worry that your friend will get angry with you, but it's better to have an angry friend...than a dead one.

Get By...With A Little Help
From Your Friends

Hopefully these stories will inspire you to TAKE ACTION—and not let friendships ruin you, drag you down, or make things worse. There is a lot of pain out there—it's easy to find. But at the same time, there are a lot of awesome people out there who *will* support and love you, regardless of your issues—or theirs. We hope that you will find them, and that you'll find it within yourself to be a good friend to them. A truly good friend is worth holding onto!

CHAPTER 7

CRAZY IN LOVE
Relationships and Mental Health

"If I lay here, If I just lay here, would you lie with me and just forget the world?"

—Snow Patrol, "Chasing Cars"

ROSS *I definitely had a long learning curve in terms of relationships and bipolar disorder. In high school, I was so massively affected by the mood swings, the anger, and psychosis that I didn't have any romantic relationships. I didn't have my first real relationship until I was 19. I had no clue how to deal with bipolar disorder or the way I felt about myself. My* *mood dictated the way I would treat my girlfriend. On good days, she got flowers, candy, cards, gifts. On bad days, I called her ridiculous names and went out of my way to hurt her. Not surprisingly, that relationship ended after only six months, when I cheated on her.*

My next relationship lasted for 10 months, and in a lot of ways, was even worse than the first one. I dated a girl who also had some mental health issues of her own. In this relationship, I was able to take all the focus off of me, and project all of the lack of caring and concern I should have had for myself—into caring for her. Looking back, I can clearly see how much pain I was in and how willing I was to push it aside to focus my energies on someone else. I took all of her abuse, and eventually she broke up with me. I held onto the idea of that relationship for a long time. It took me probably two years before I dated anyone seriously again. Even after the breakup, I believed she had been "the one." I had convinced myself that I needed her in my life. In retrospect, I can see now that the way I felt about myself at that time had a big impact in terms of my wanting to hold onto someone who clearly wasn't good for me, but if anyone had said as much to me back then, I would have thought they were wrong.

I grew and learned an immense amount in my next relationship. At one point we were even engaged, but we realized soon after that it wasn't going to work out. When we agreed to break up, I reverted to some of my old coping mechanisms for a night of drinking, smoking, and destruction. But when I woke up the next morning, I realized I didn't want to go back to handling things that way. Eventually I got myself to a healthy place where I could see that the breakup with my fiancée was ultimately a good thing for me. I learned so much about myself from that relationship, because it was the first one where I was able to maintain that balance of caring about myself, being there for the other person, and allowing that other person to be there for me. Don't get me wrong, the relationship had its share of problems, but I was willing to take what I had learned from it and move forward.

For a while, I swore off the idea of another long-term relationship or the possibility of finding a deep love. But then, just five months after the breakup, I went out to Los Angeles to visit my brother. While I was there, I made plans to see a friend who I had known for a while. We went out one night, the next night, and then another. The experience was surreal. It was suddenly as if we shared the same mind and could finish each other's thoughts. While she didn't have a mental disorder, she could relate to my pain enough to where she could provide the comfort I so desperately needed. My love for her grew so quickly that I was almost afraid it was related to a manic high. But that thought faded when I got back home to DC and realized that this was a different type of connection—one I had never had before—because I had never been open to something so healthy. We dated long distance for a year, then I moved out to L.A., and we have been together now for five years.

When we first moved in together, I fully realized the damage left from my past relationships. To deal with my disorder, I had created a serious wall around myself, and no one could scale it. There was no way of fully recognizing this when I lived on my own. But my girlfriend worked with me and gradually helped me to feel comfortable letting down my walls, so I could be open to new experiences that were safe. I can sometimes feel a lot of anxiety in certain social settings. But with her help, I was able to become more confident and comfortable around other people. She also helped me to better manage my anger, which often used to explode (and still can sometimes) for little or no reason. She was patient and tried to help me identify what was happening before I would flip out. But this didn't happen overnight. She is probably the most patient and loving person I know, and of course it takes a lot of work from my end too. I am still in treatment, but having a strong, stable relationship in my life has been a huge help to me as well.

That Lovin' Feeling

You know that feeling...you meet someone new, and suddenly you find you can't stop thinking about this person. As you go through your day, no matter what you may encounter, your face is plastered with a conspicuous perma-grin. When you think about this new person in your life your body tingles. And whenever you're together, the feeling intensifies. Your perceptions sharpen. The sky looks bluer, and the trees greener (even in the dead of winter). You have boundless energy. Everything seems better.

At the start of a relationship, most people are on their best behavior. They do everything they can to make the euphoria last. As Chris Rock says, when you start dating someone new, no one leads with all of their baggage. I mean really, who wants to know that you have a stalker? Or that your last relationship ended because you cheated on your girlfriend? Or that you don't typically believe in commitment for more than two weeks at a time? Sometimes people wait to discuss the heavy things.

Eventually, the initial intense feelings of "love" may fade. If and when they do, you're bound to question the reason. Maybe it was just a moment in time. Maybe it was real, or maybe it had just been some odd combination of alcohol and happiness. Whatever the explanation, when love disappears, it can feel utterly devastating, especially if it signifies the end of a long relationship with someone who you felt had really understood you. Breakups can do fascinating things to your self-esteem. In the worst-case scenario, they can leave mental scars that can take what seems like an eternity to heal. Or alternatively, they can also help you to discover new and exciting things about yourself.

We all know of someone who never quite got over a certain relationship. She still holds onto the possibility that she and her partner will one day get back together, even if the relationship was unhealthy or ended some years ago. Personal connections are painful to relinquish. Sometimes people just don't know how to move on, as much as they may want to.

Love Hurts: Surviving A Breakup

Plain and simple, breakups *suck*. To say that they're painful is a serious understatement. It doesn't just hurt—it can feel almost like someone literally reached into your chest and pulled out your heart. It can feel brutal, as though life can't get any worse. You walk around oozing pain and suffering from the inside out. Everything aches. And in the beginning, there looks to be no end in sight.

If you have a mental disorder, your recovery from a breakup can be especially hard to manage. For some people who have already been diagnosed with a mental disorder, a major life change like a breakup can cause an episode to reoccur. Or it can bring to the surface a mental disorder that you've been refusing to acknowledge, forcing you to deal with it.

It's completely natural to experience pain after a breakup, but for some, that heartache will go a step further and lead to depression. In order to be diagnosed with clinical depression, you have to have exhibited the following symptoms for two to three weeks:

- A persistent sad, anxious or empty mood

- Decreased energy, feeling constantly tired

- Not finding pleasure in anything

- Loss of sex drive

- Difficulty concentrating or making decisions

- Insomnia, waking up too early or oversleeping

- Weight gain or loss

- Feelings of guilt, worthlessness, helplessness

- Excessive crying

- Thoughts of death or suicide

It's important for us to distinguish between feeling "depressed," and actually suffering from (clinical) *depression*. There is a real difference between the two. When you *feel* depressed, there is a cause—maybe you had a bad day, or you just received some bad news. It's painful and you're unhappy, yes—but as time passes, you start to feel better. *Depression* as a mental disorder is something different. "The blues" last for weeks or even longer, and it isn't tied to any one single piece of bad news or to having a difficult day. Time passes, but you still don't heal. It's not a passing mood—you *can't* make yourself feel better. *You need help.* The best way to determine whether or not you are clinically depressed is to visit a mental health professional and explain your situation. With the right treatment, the majority of those who seek help *do* get better—and many start to feel better in just a few short weeks.

EMILY suffers from both depression and anorexia. *The day my boyfriend broke up with me, I literally felt like I was going to die. After the breakup, things got even worse. My weight plummeted. My grades tanked. I literally couldn't leave my house or get out of bed (except to go to the bathroom) for weeks. My best friend dragged me to the doctor after I got a bad flu, but really it was more of a forced intervention. She took me in for a prescription for antibiotics, but I came out with a diagnosis of depression and anorexia. There was no pill strong enough to take away my pain. I flirted with the idea of taking medication for the depression, but at the time I was convinced that I'd never fully get through it unless I could literally feel my pain. It was like I had been numb to my deepest self, while also crying every day. It was very strange and almost impossible to put into words. But once I finally came to terms with* *the fact that I was clinically depressed, I wanted to feel every tear, process every moment. I was afraid that if I didn't, it would stay with me forever.*

It's been six years since Emily was diagnosed with depression. She still has her issues, and she's relapsed a few times, but now she's aware of herself enough to know what she has to do to maintain her health.

It can be hard to seek help for a mental disorder at any point in life, but even more difficult after a breakup. You may not want the other person to feel they have that power over you. Or you may feel even worse about yourself—thinking that your boyfriend or girlfriend wouldn't have left if you weren't a terrible person. But the truth is, for most people, it's not the actual *loss* of a person or of a relationship that triggers an emotional episode—it's the *change.* Change of any kind can be hard to handle when you have a mental disorder. And the change resulting from a broken relationship should be treated like any other major life change—you need to monitor yourself and your moods, educate yourself about ways in which change can affect your disorder, and most importantly—make it a priority to seek the help you need.

A Dangerous Bond

Let's say you've met someone you like very much. She really looks at you when you're talking, as if she can see through you. You feel exposed, yet somehow accepted. As you spend more time with her, you feel yourself standing at the precipice, opening your mouth and falling through the void. It's scary, but you feel you can take the risk. You share your story, and strangely, she doesn't run away from you, screaming. She understands. She just "gets it"—both you *and* your issue. Why? Because *she* has that same issue, too. This commonality can forge a very powerful bond.

We already covered some of this in chapter six when we talked about friendships, but it's a totally different thing when dealing with a love interest. In sharing with such a person—someone who is able to bond with you about a certain mental health issue—your vulnerability reaches a new level, and the rush of emotions is powerful. You feel complete, and almost relieved. You've hidden your feelings for so long, yearning for someone to understand you, and finally it seems your wish has come true. You're liberated from the burden of having to hide your unhealthy thoughts and behaviors, because now you have a partner in crime. But this is where you need to be careful—this is where the relationship can get complicated.

Many people bond in the midst of serious dysfunction. These ties can be deep and profound. There's a lot at stake—the relationship allows you to behave in all the old, unhealthy ways that are so familiar and comforting. Your girlfriend, boyfriend, lover, significant other, becomes your enabler. He or she lets your disorder *thrive*. And who doesn't love their enablers?

This is a dangerous relationship—and it happens all the time. If neither person in the relationship confronts their disorders, it can create an environment that breeds even more self-destruction. Now, any feelings of worthlessness you may have already had related to your disorder are potentially reinforced by the relationship and this new "love." You feel as if this person is the only one who knows the real you, the damaged you—and he or she perpetuates the notion that you're only capable of being damaged for life. The patterns you developed of hating yourself actually get strengthened.

There is absolutely nothing wrong with being in a relationship with someone who has a mental disorder, even if you have one yourself. But it can also be tricky. Your relationship will have a greater chance of success if you make a focused attempt to work on your issues together. Otherwise you run the risk of accumulating years of anger, guilt and fear, which could sabotage your best intentions for maintaining your own health – while also threatening your future as a couple.

You Hate Me, I Hate Me

Let's say you're in a relationship that isn't working. You want to leave, you know that you should, but you stay—for fear of being alone. So you find ways to rationalize his anger. His outbursts. His horrible, demeaning comments. All the times he embarrasses you in public. Cheats on you. Goes out of his way to hurt you. You start to believe you may even deserve it—that you're pathetic and unworthy of love. You begin to feel lucky just to have *someone* who will stay with you, so you continue to take it. The negative comments. The lack of attention. The pain. The black eyes. You routinely give everything but get nothing in return—and all the while, thinking that it's somehow your fault.

One of the largest and most common by-products of mental disorders (or traumatic life events) can be *self-hate*. If you hate yourself and you're in a relationship, then you're particularly vulnerable to emotional or physical abuse—as the victim or the perpetrator. But this balance of power *can* change. If you can identify that you need to get out, you *can* do it. It may take time and a lot of work, but if you can relate on any level to this sort of situation, something is seriously wrong. *You need to seek help immediately.*

ANGELA was 18 when she got out of a negative relationship that she had been in for four years. *The hardest thing for me to do was leave him, and no one else could understand why. He treated me like absolute crap. He never acted like he cared about me, and seemed to constantly go out of his way to hurt me. It's weird to say, but even after we broke up, I held onto him emotionally for over two years. It was only after I learned more about ME—that I realized how he had represented every negative thought I had about myself.*

Subconsciously, most individuals are likely to seek out relationships that validate the beliefs they have about themselves—good or bad. For example, if you have a mental health issue and if you're full of self-hate, it's difficult for you to enter a relationship with someone who truly cherishes you. Your partner may tell you the wonderful things she or he loves about you, but if you're gripped by self-hate, the words and concepts will feel too foreign for you to accept. You may be so accustomed to hearing the opposite—either because you consistently tell yourself that you're worthless, or because someone has abused you—that you actually *push away the love.* You may push so hard that ultimately you lose the person, the one who really wanted to love you. Or maybe you act out, scaring off the new person without meaning to, causing him or her to treat you differently—maybe even badly—since that's what you're used to.

This applies to more than just romantic relationships. With friends, family members, classmates, teammates, or anyone in your life—the way you think of yourself will absolutely shape the way you respond to others. For example, you may think you're stupid, despite your *A+* average, academic awards, and Herculean vocabulary. No matter what anyone tells you, you're afraid people will one day learn "the truth" about you—the "stupid," "no-good," "worthless" you. If you truly believe this, then whenever people try to tell you otherwise, it won't register. You'll disregard the compliments entirely, while seeking to confirm your stupidity. You may tell yourself that people who see good things in you are all wrong, that they don't really know what goes on inside you. Maybe you go over and over mistakes you have made, or bring to mind all the times when anyone called you stupid—anything to cling to the old, negative, familiar view of yourself.

This happens to a lot of people, but that doesn't mean that you're destined to sabotage your life by living out your anxieties. By identifying and understanding your beliefs about yourself, you will give yourself a compass that can help you navigate your life. If you're prone to feeling worthless, then knowing that about yourself is the first step toward getting over it. *Self-awareness is key.*

It's no different with romantic relationships. If you are inclined toward abusive ones, you need to know that you are not alone, but that you *can* change these patterns. Identify your self-hate, or the beliefs you have about yourself that make it acceptable (in your mind) for people to treat you badly. Get into it. Where does this come from? Why do you believe this about yourself? Who was the first person who made you feel this way? Knowing this will help you come to terms with the truth about yourself, which is half the battle.

However, it's only the first step in what may be a lifelong process. If you're looking to end a destructive relationship, we implore you to seek help. You do have an out, but you may need some time to muster the strength to leave, develop a support system, and identify a safe place to go. But most importantly, you have to be the one to make the decision. Nobody can force you to leave an unhealthy relationship. Only *you* can do it. And *you can*.

How Do I Tell The Person I Love About My Disorder?

Telling a boyfriend or girlfriend that you have a mental disorder can be really hard. Most people wonder what will happen if they disclose something so personal. Would it be better to stay silent? Would it be easier to pretend everything is fine? Maybe it has been so long since you last loved someone that you are afraid to sabotage it. Maybe the last time you told someone about your disorder, that person couldn't handle it and walked away. Or maybe you've never told anyone, let alone the person you love. Regardless of your situation, if you feel it's time to open up, you have options.

Before you say anything, it may help to talk with a mental health professional. You will probably be dealing with a lot of

How Do I Tell My Partner About My Problems?

- Have the support of your friends and/or family. You need someone you can talk to about the experience, and who can help you process your feelings.

- Try to talk to your boyfriend or girlfriend about this in a natural way. Don't assault them with it.

- Don't say negative things about yourself while discussing the situation. Be confident and hold yourself in a positive light.

- Be honest. Speak straightforwardly about your disorder or what you have been through.

- Don't panic if the first reaction is negative. Realize that when someone hears this for the first time, it may be a shock. His response may be an initial gut reaction, and not a true reflection of how he will feel once he's given it some thought—or how he may feel about it in the future.

- Be willing to educate your partner about your disorder. Explain that most mental disorders have a high treatment rate.

- Be clear about how your disorder or experience may or may not change the relationship. Tell your partner what you may need from her. But don't expect too much at first. She may need some time to process this new information.

- Let your partner know you did not choose to have a mental disorder. You are not seeking attention. You are doing everything you can to be healthy, which is why you are telling the person you love.

- Be open to questions about the disorder and the experience.

- Give the person time. And REMAIN CONFIDENT. Do not make your partner the key to your happiness or future. You were fine before this person came along, and you'll be okay again if it doesn't work out.

> • Be prepared for any kind of reaction. The person may not be emotionally equipped to handle it well. He could flip out, calling you every name imaginable and reinforcing your worst fears. Or, he might calmly thank you for being honest, just before he then lets you know that he wants out of the relationship. He could ask for time to consider what you've said. Or, best-case scenario, he could completely empathize and want to understand, opening up a new level of the relationship.

fears and emotions. You may be afraid that your boyfriend or girlfriend will judge you, embarrass you, not understand you, or possibly even leave. Those are real fears, and talking with a doctor or counselor can help you to face them. Once you understand the emotions that are driving you, you can discuss ways to tell your boyfriend or girlfriend that you have a mental disorder. Educating yourself about your disorder is the best way to increase your confidence.

When you're finally ready to talk to your partner about your disorder, you need to be prepared for anything. But remember the things your mental health professional may have suggested to help yourself feel more comfortable, and that taking this important step is the best thing for both of you in the long run. Then, plunge in.

You Will Love Again: Staying Positive After A Breakup

All of these reactions are possible, but you have to stay strong in the belief that someone who really loves you will accept you for who you are. If someone can't handle the truth about your mental disorder, the relationship probably didn't have much of a future anyway. That may be hard to hear, especially when someone leaves or hurts you because of something that's beyond your control. Hopefully, you have other support from friends, family, or someone who can be there to help you cope if your partner abandons you.

It can be traumatic and difficult to regain stability after experiencing such a loss. As we have stressed throughout this book, it can also lead to a relapse with a disorder, so whenever you're faced with such an emotionally intense situation, don't feel like you have to brave it on your own. Talk to a mental health professional, your friends, your family, and take every step possible to avoid going through another major episode. Also remember that breakups can oftentimes be for the best. They can even be a good way for you to learn more about yourself and what it is that you really need from a relationship. Of course it doesn't feel like that right after you've just heard the words, "I don't think we should see each other any more." But if you give it time and manage to get the help you need, you *will* survive, and eventually move on to bigger and better things.

If You Are Worried About Your Boyfriend/Girlfriend

Maybe your problem isn't telling someone you love that you have a disorder. Maybe it's *the person you love* who's behaving strangely. It may start slowly. You notice your boyfriend doing things he never did before or your girlfriend neglecting things she used to enjoy. When you hug her, she seems a little thinner. When he drinks, he gets really angry. You try to rationalize it, telling yourself it's "normal," that everyone has their demons. But then you wake up in the middle of the night to find her crying. Or when he's drunk, he opens up to you about things like a death, a divorce, or thoughts about wanting to kill himself. He has blackouts. She says it's just a phase. "It's not that big of a deal." "You worry too much." "Everything is fine..."

But deep down, you know something isn't right. The changes in behavior continue. Now, she's not just a little thinner, she's emaciated. He isn't just angry, he's punching holes in walls. You worried that this was coming, but you didn't want to believe it was possible. So now what do you do?

MARIA tried to learn more about her boyfriend's extreme mood swings. *I noticed a lot of strange changes in my boyfriend's behavior. He went from confident and talkative, to withdrawn and having no interest in anything. He stopped wanting to see his friends, didn't want to see me, and his moods became totally unpredictable. I read some stuff online, and then went to the counseling center to talk to someone. I needed to try to understand why this was happening. All I knew is that it wasn't normal, and that it scared me.*

Approaching a boyfriend or girlfriend in this situation can be intimidating. You may be afraid of the consequences, but eventually it gets to the point where you can no longer live in denial. There are some steps you can take to make this process easier.

Taking these steps will not guarantee that the person you love will want to listen to you. She may feel defiant, exposed, angry, or scared. Reassure her that you care—that you only want the best for her—and will be there to help her through the process.

And that process can be a long one. You may fear that you could lose things about the person that you love. But love can help you to hang in there and work through it. Some people with less severe disorders may find the right treatment quickly. For others, it may take years. Regardless, throughout the process, it will be important to talk with the person about what he or she may or may not need from you. Have this conversation as soon and as frequently as possible. It can

How Do I Prepare for Telling My Boyfriend/Girlfriend That I'm Worried?

- Educate yourself on your boyfriend or girlfriend's symptoms by reading books, going online, and any way you can to learn about their disorder.

- Learn about the warning signs of various disorders.

- Find out what types of things can bring out the disorder or lead to relapses.

- Read about available treatments for the disorder.

- Think about what it must be like for them to experience the symptoms of their disorder.

help the person feel more comfortable about having the disorder, while also enabling you to grow closer to one another.

Much like with families, you will need to find a balance between empowering and enabling the person with the disorder. Just because someone is sick does not mean that he or she has the right to dominate the relationship. You also have needs, and they don't go away, especially not because someone you love has a mental disorder. Remember to take care of yourself, too.

Deciding to End An Unhealthy Relationship

If you're in a relationship with someone who refuses to seek help for their problems, remember that there are limits to what you can do. You can talk to a professional, call a hotline or go to a series of websites to explore your options. But if a person is not open to seeking help, you cannot force, persuade, or manipulate him or her into doing it. The person may agree to go along with your request, just to have you stop nagging them—but this isn't an effective way to get treatment for a mental disorder. Unless a person truly wants to be helped, your chances of seeing lasting change will be slim to none.

When your attempts to help or understand are rejected, it hurts. It's confusing. It can make you want to abandon the relationship, and you may ultimately decide to do so. You sit there hoping that one day you'll break down the walls and the storm will end, but deep down, you're afraid it never will. If this is the case, your best option is to find a mental health professional and start talking. You also need to look out for *yourself.* If you allow your own mental health to slide, you'll have very little to give to anyone else. You could even end up worse than your partner. You can regain your health, but first you have to identify and talk about the problem. And *this*, you can do.

The decision to leave can become even more complicated if both of you have a mental disorder or problem. Some of the best relationships are the result of two people learning how to be healthy together. Unfortunately, it can also be common for one person to relapse. The fear of commitment can be a trigger for a relapse, and there may be others. No matter what the trigger, the person who didn't slip may find it easy to go back into a destructive mode, so be sure to take care of yourself if you're in this situation.

Whether or not to leave is your decision—no one can make it for you. Some people try to stick it out, but if nothing changes, they end up living in bad relationships for years. Other people need to cut the cord and move on with their lives. There's no right or wrong—you just have to do what is right for you. But whatever you do, remember the person with whom you're breaking up might be devastated. So do try to be as loving as possible, even as you're leaving.

Leaving someone you love is a big decision, one not to be taken lightly. Talking to someone about your situation will enable you to make a sound choice about what to do. But if you hear manipulative, desperate or unhealthy comments from your partner like, "I will die if you leave," you need to remember that *your partner's life is not your responsibility.* You can try to get them the help they need, but when someone makes the fateful choice to take his or her life, know that there is much more going on there than just one tumultuous relationship. You cannot—under any circumstances—allow yourself to take the blame.

JOSE was 19 when he felt he needed to break up with his girlfriend, but he was afraid about what might happen to her. *My girlfriend and I were about to separate for good, but then she told me that she would kill herself if we broke up. I didn't know what to do. I obviously didn't want her to die, but I also didn't want to be in the relationship anymore. This dragged on like this for months. Finally, I went to see a counselor on campus. Eventually we worked out a plan that allowed me to deal with the situation while also protecting her. But let me tell you, it was not easy. I don't know if I would have even gotten through it without the help of a counselor.*

Breakups are powerful events in a person's life. One of the top reasons that Ross is asked to speak to a high school or college is when the school is dealing with the traumatic aftermath of a student's suicide. A suicide, which—not surprisingly—is usually tied in some way to a breakup. And it typically goes something like this: boy meets girl, they fall in love, girl dumps boy, boy takes his own life. But remember, 90% of all people who take their own lives *already have* a mental disorder, aside from the suicidal thoughts. Most experts agree that a breakup is never solely responsible for a suicide. It's profoundly more complicated than that. If someone is filled with self-hate and shame, a relationship may be the only positive thing in his or her life—but that still doesn't mean that the loss of that relationship directly inspired the person's suicide. The breakup didn't create the feelings of self-hate, and the relationship could not have fixed or changed those feelings. Just because a person breaks up with someone who then goes on to commit suicide, that person is **not** responsible.

That said, if you are dating someone who continually talks about suicide—especially **if they have a specific plan**—then you must tell someone you trust. As we said in chapter six, if the person has a plan, then you must take action. Devising a suicide plan is typically the last step someone takes before attempting to take his or her own life. If you ever find yourself in this situation, call a suicide hotline **immediately** and find out what you can do. We have included several emergency numbers for you in the back of this book.

(It's also important to note that not every person who attempts to take his or her own life actually has a plan, or they may not discuss it. So the general rule of thumb is that *anytime* you feel someone may be experiencing any type of mental disorder—whether you know the person to be suicidal or not—you should encourage them to seek help.)

Even the most successful relationships can be hard enough. Mental health issues only heighten the drama. But if you make real efforts to take care of yourself, they can be rewarding and satisfying. Always remember, you are not alone. Finding out what you can do to help yourself and your partner deal with a disorder will be of great benefit to you— not only in this relationship, but it will help you to be better equipped to deal with these things in the future.

Moving Beyond Your Scars

When you've been involved in a relationship or a breakup with someone who has a disorder, it may seem that things will never get better. Let us assure you that the pain will pass. The younger you are, the harder it is to believe this—but with time, things do change. And with every experience, you will grow stronger (and hopefully, wiser).

ALISON discovered that she was in a relationship with someone who could not support her emotionally as she grieved the loss of her brother. *Eventually, she broke up with him. I was so scared. My brother died, and then I lost my boyfriend. I felt like a girl who was losing every man in her life. So as I embarked on my grieving, I made two rules for myself: no drinking alcohol and no men. I felt totally out of control. I had no reason to "celebrate" anything.*

Eventually I did start dating again, but I had difficulty allowing myself to be vulnerable. I felt there was no way anyone on my campus could understand my grief, and I was even more certain that no one would want to. I was sure that if anyone expressed interest in me, they obviously didn't know what they were getting themselves into—and if they did, they wouldn't want anything to do with me.

Five years after my brother's death, I found myself longing for a relationship. I started dating a guy who was fairly emo-

tional and was dealing with a lot of his own personal issues. I will say that he understood what it was like to wallow in pain, but after the first few months of getting into a very emotionally intertwined relationship with him, I realized I needed more. I needed someone who not only could "handle" my emotions, but someone who challenged me, could make me laugh, and who made me look forward to the future. Being with this person just kept me stuck in my grief.

Once I came to appreciate what I had to offer in a relationship and what else defined me, I started to seek out people who could fulfill all of my needs—emotional, intellectual, playful. I began a relationship with a well-rounded guy who lets me grieve, makes me laugh, and makes me think. And now that I see what I have to offer—that there is more to me than just my grief—I can provide him with what he needs, as well.

A therapist I went to after my brother died told me that my next big struggle would come when I entered my next serious relationship. With my experiences as a suicide survivor, she said that I might have attachment issues and could inherently push away anyone close to me, as I would subconsciously be afraid of losing them. In the past six years since losing my brother, I have spent a great deal of time discovering who I am and what my experiences have meant to me. Now that I have found someone I can see a possible future with, I have been able to pursue this relationship like any other twentysomething. Attachment issues are nowhere to be found; I have a healthy view of relationships and friendships, and I know that while I am forever changed by what happened, I don't have to be forever identified by the loss of my brother.

Past events in our lives can leave scars. Deep ones. Even if no one else can see the marks, we feel them profoundly. When we first attempt to find someone to love after such an event, the event itself may be all we can think about. Some people will try to ignore the trauma of what happened, believing it doesn't really affect them. They may enter into unhealthy situations. Some will latch on at the first sign of caring, others will laugh at the idea that anyone *could* care, and many will remain distant, wondering if their emotional scars will ever heal.

When you don't know how to deal with your own grief, it's easy to get into a relationship with someone who is stuck in the same place. Eventually you realize that you're trapped in an unhealthy relationship. Some people see this and try to get out, while others revel in the pain.

As we mentioned, it takes time to work through these issues. Having the support of family and friends is instrumental to the healing process. If you are having attachment issues as a result of a death, your parents' divorce, abuse, a mental disorder, or some other issue, remember—no matter how scared you may be of losing someone, you can also become stronger. You don't have to live with the scars forever. And you *don't* have to let pain and loss rule your life.

Love Lifts Us Up

Love takes work. Most of us hope to one day find the ideal person to complement us or make our lives easier. Every day there are millions of stories about love in magazines, books, blogs, and everything imaginable—and almost all of them focus on the hope we all share of ultimately finding this person. Love can be the most powerful force any of us will ever experience.

Your boyfriend or girlfriend can't be your therapist or your psychologist. Much like a good friend, though, they can work with you to help make you stronger. But your disorder can get out of control at times, and your partner may not always know what to do. Hopefully, you can identify and work on these things with your partner as well as your therapist.

It's also important not to make your disorder the focus of your relationship. Ross and his girlfriend have worked on maintaining his mental health, but his disorder isn't the sum of their relationship. They are both well aware of his triggers and work hard on communication. He also knows that not every disagreement or negative experience is a direct result of his disorder.

ROSS *It has taken a long time to identify what is and isn't connected to the disorder, but we are doing a good job. My girlfriend also has bad days and tough things to deal with, which is when I need to be able to be present for her. When she is going through a rough time, I work hard to not put the focus on me.*

The Power of Commitment

A lot of people have given up on long-term relationships in favor of "friends with benefits," one-night stands, the casual

How Can I Help Our Relationship Work Well for Both of Us?

- Keep the lines of communication open with your boyfriend or girlfriend.

- Learn to identify what things happen as a result of your disorder as opposed to things that are just regular life occurrences, and what you can do to deal with both.

- Know your limits and when you should consult with your mental health professional.

- Work with your psychologist or therapist to remove those things that make it difficult for you to be close to others. And if you are in a relationship that can help you, then work to find ways for that to continue.

- Find a balance. Don't make the relationship revolve entirely around you or your disorder.

hookup. We hear a lot of stories about not having time for a relationship, not wanting to deal with the drama, not being able to find the "perfect" person, and other much more superficial reasons for passing on commitment. But a successful long-term relationship can be a beautiful thing and add stability, strength, and support to all areas of your life.

Whether or not you have a mental disorder, don't give up on the idea of love or long-term relationships. You can't always predict when your ideal match is going to come along, but try to remain open to the possibility! The more positive you are about love—and about *yourself*—the better your chances of finding a successful relationship in the future.

CRAZY IN LOVE

Love is a wonderful thing, but when you add a mental disorder to the mix, sometimes all bets are off. That's not to say that long-term relationships under these circumstances are impossible, but they can take even more effort. As a result, however, you could also end up building an even stronger and more resilient bond with your partner. Continue to learn as much as you can about each other, have patience, and enjoy the process.

CONCLUSION

In 2005, author Gail Griffith was speaking at the Active Minds National Conference when she told an audience of college students, "*YOU will be the generation that removes this stigma!*" It's a powerful statement about mental health—and one with a lot of meaning. If you're in high school or college, then it was your parents' generation that removed the stigma surrounding cancer. It was your grandparents' generation that was there during the Civil Rights movement. Your great grandparents fought in World War II, and your great-great grandparents were around when women were first given the right to vote. But what will distinguish YOUR generation? *Will yours be the generation that finally removes the painful stigma surrounding mental disorders?* We certainly hope so.

None of us chose to live with this stigma. It has been passed down for hundreds of years—from our grandparents, to our parents, and now to us. We didn't choose to live in a world where people talk *about* each other, instead of *to* each other. A world where it is more acceptable to have a friend who gets wasted than it is to have a friend who openly shows emotion. A world where you are made to feel afraid or ashamed, every single day, about the very thoughts and emotions that make you the unique individual you are! We didn't choose to live in a world like this, but we *can* choose to end these unnecessary stereotypes, once and for all. We have to. Otherwise we risk losing more friends, or maybe even losing ourselves.

If you worry that maybe this stigma won't go away—that maybe everything connected with the understanding of mental disorders will remain the same, or grow even worse over the next 10 years—then you have to take action. A lot of people may sit around feeling helpless, as if there is nothing they can do. Not true. You may not be able to single-handedly fix this problem across the board, but you can absolutely make the effort to STOP THE STIGMA in your personal life—among your friends, and among your family. And it's worth it to try, for the sake of everyone close to you.

If you are going to make this effort to encourage change, it is going to take an immense amount of strength. Remember, when women stood up and asked for the right to vote, they were mocked, labeled as terrorists, and some were even jailed. When Martin Luther King Jr. and other brave activists wanted equal rights, they risked their lives to get them. You won't have to endure exactly what these people did, but you will have to be prepared to deal with others who may label you as "weak," "oversensitive," "stupid," and a host of other ridiculous, baseless names. However, real weakness is identifying a problem and then not doing a thing about it. Weakness is seeing people all around you with mental health issues who are suffering this stigma, and staying silent. Or worse—falling victim to this stereotyping yourself. The real weakness is in *not* changing.

It's time for all of us to stand up, and STOP ACCEPTING THE OLD WAYS OF DEALING with mental health issues. It's time for us to STOP LOSING THE LIVES of our friends, our families, the people we care most about, simply because of needless stigma and lack of understanding. It's time for all of us to STOP LOSING...*PERIOD.* It's time to START WINNING the campaign of many...for a sound mind! The campaign to let every generation feel that they have the right to talk about their needs and emotions.

We hope you have found comfort and empowerment through the words in this book, and that you will turn to it as a resource whenever you need information, or even just a reminder that *you're not alone.* We hope it has left you with a better understanding of mental disorders and what it means to have a mental health issue, and that these are not things of which you should ever have to feel ashamed.

Finally, we hope you will have the strength to use the experience and knowledge of those who came before you—to help make life better for those who come after you. It's time we all learned that each of us has a *right*—and a *responsibility*—to face our issues, be honest about our needs and emotions, and most importantly, to ask for help when we need it.

So here's to putting on your REAL happy face...get out there and start living the life you know you want. You deserve it. *Take charge of your mental health!*

EPILOGUE

ROSS SZABO *When I turned 21, my parents took me out to dinner. At one point they both started crying. They told me there was a time when they were afraid I wouldn't even live to be 21. As I sit here now at 29, looking back at the life I've lived to this point, I am so thankful. I am not necessarily thankful for having bipolar disorder, because even though I'm able to deal with it now, there was a long time when I wasn't. My parents tell me I have the same personality now that I did when I was a child—that they had watched that side of me disappear during my darkest days with the disorder (from about ages 15 to 23). That is one of the many reasons why I believe this disorder doesn't define who I am. But it took me a long time to learn that. There were so many days of my life where my parents, friends and I were all hoping that the person we once knew would just come back. In the end, I can't attribute my fortune in finally finding a way to deal with this monster to any one thing. However, I can say that the ways in which I learned to deal with this disorder have greatly enhanced my family, friendships, and other relationships. For that much, I am thankful.*

Traveling around the country and speaking has been the most rewarding and fascinating opportunity I could have ever imag-

ined. *I have eaten the local cuisines in over 40 states, visited every major city, and spent countless hours viewing this country from the sky, even to the point where I now know the normal landing patterns at all the major airports! I have driven most of the roads. I have met some amazing people, both young and old, through which I've made a lot of friends. I have felt the warm embrace of young men and women as they wholeheartedly thanked me or cried on my shoulder, lamenting feelings of hopelessness. I've heard endless stories of what mental disorders can do to individuals, families, and friends. I have seen a lot of really great programs in hundreds of inspiring schools and communities. Overall, I have seen that, beyond the politics, the talking heads and the news, at the heart of this issue are thousands of people working tirelessly—to educate others about mental health—and make this country better.*

I have been humbled in ways that have truly connected me to humanity. I wish I could share every story with you, but one in particular definitely stands out in my mind. I was speaking at a mental health conference at George Washington University in Washington DC. Throughout my presentation, I noticed that a deaf and blind man was in my audience. He had two translators. The first knew sign language to give to the other translator, and the second translator would actually sign into the man's hands, so that he could understand what was being said. I assumed he went blind later in life so that he knew sign language, but then still had to learn to communicate via someone signing into his hands. After my presentation, he asked a question related to pop culture, and I was amazed that he was so familiar with everything. After questions and answers, the man approached me with his translators. He thanked me for speaking out about these issues in a positive way because he had been through so many negative things in his life, and didn't need to hear the negative anymore. He said that it was nice to know someone understood his pain. I asked his translators to show me how to say "you're welcome" to the man. As I signed the phrase into his hands, he began to cry. In all the years I have been doing this work, I have cried maybe three times in front of other people (possibly a million other times in private), and that was certainly one of those times. We shared a few emotional moments together, then hugged and said our goodbyes.

As I walked out to my car later that day, I thought about the 17-year-old boy who had suffered so much, and who was once terrified to stand up in front of his classroom. And how I managed to get where I am today. Thankfully I was taught from a young age to stand up for myself and for others who weren't being treated fairly. My parents instilled this belief in me, not just because it is noble, but because it is right.

I know that without my disorder, I would not have had the opportunity to have so many of the incredible experiences I've had over the years. I also know that my disorder will be with me—for better or worse—for the rest of my life. I can only hope that the voice I gained at age 17 and all that I've learned since the first days of this disorder will continue to help me in my own life—as well as provide a voice, a positive example, and HOPE to all the people I continue to reach.

RESOURCES
and Ways to Get Involved

If you or someone you know may be suffering from a mental disorder, please refer to the following list of websites, organizations and suggested reading. There is a wealth of information out there, and many people who are available to help you to cope and to learn more about certain mental health issues. Please remember that you may also research additional mental health resources that may be available in your local community.

Crisis Numbers

Please note these numbers if you or a loved one is in need of IMMEDIATE HELP:

Knowledge Exchange Network (KEN)
1-800-789-2647 or
1-877-495-0009
Live operators available 8:30 AM – 5:00 PM EST to refer you to public mental health clinics in your area.

American Psychological Association
Public Education Line
1-800-964-2000

Live operators available to help you 24/7 and refer you to local APA board certified psychologists.

RESOURCES

American Psychiatric Association Answer Center
(202) 682-6000

Live operators available 24/7 to refer you to local APA board certified psychiatrists.

1-800-THERAPIST
1-800-843-7274

Live counselors 9 AM – 5 PM will refer you to various mental health professionals near you.

National Hopeline Network
1-800-SUICIDE
(1-800-784-2433)

Live certified counselors available 24/7 to help those in immediate distress.

American Mental Health Counselors Association/
ProvisionsConsulting
1-877-956-6400

A toll-free, national find-a-therapist referral service.

National Suicide Prevention Hotline
1-800-273-TALK (8255)

Counselors available 24/7 for referrals.

Mental Disorder Resources

Please refer to the following list for help and information regarding specific mental disorders.

Anxiety Disorders

Anxiety Disorders Association of America
8730 Georgia Ave., Suite 600
Silver Spring, MD 20910
(240) 485-1001
www.adaa.org

Attention Deficit/Hyperactivity Disorder

Children and Adults with Attention Deficit/Hyperactivity Disorder
8181 Professional Place, Suite 150
Landover, MD 20785
1-800-233-4050
www.chadd.org

Bipolar Disorder and Depression

Child and Adolescent Bipolar Foundation
1000 Skokie Blvd., Suite 570
Wilmette, IL 60091
(847) 256-8525
www.bpkids.org

Depression and Bipolar Support Alliance
730 N. Franklin Street, Suite 501
Chicago, IL 60610
1-800-826-3632
www.dbsalliance.org

Depression and Related Affective Disorders Association
8201 Greensboro Drive, Suite 300
McLean, VA 22102
(703) 610-9026
www.drada.org

Eating Disorders

National Eating Disorders Association
603 Stewart St., Suite 803
Seattle, WA 98101
1-800-931-2237
www.nationaleatingdisorders.org

Renfrew Center for Eating Disorders
475 Spring Lane
Philadelphia, PA 19128
1-877-367-3383
www.renfrew.org

Schizophrenia

National Alliance for Research on Schizophrenia and Depression
60 Cutter Mill Road, Suite 404
Great Neck, NY 11021
1-800-829-8289
www.narsad.org

Suicide

American Association of Suicidology
5221 Wisconsin Avenue, NW
Washington, DC 20015
(202) 237-2280
www.suicidology.org

BehindHappyFaces.com

American Foundation for Suicide Prevention
120 Wall Street, 22nd Floor
New York, NY 10005
1-888-333-2377
www.afsp.org

Kristin Brooks Hope Center
615 7th St. NE
Washington, DC 20002
1-800-SUICIDE (784-2433)
www.hopeline.com

The Jed Foundation
583 Broadway, Suite 8B
New York, NY 10012
(212) 647-7544
www.jedfoundation.org
www.ulifeline.org

National Organization for People of Color Against Suicide
4715 Sargent Rd., NE
Washington, DC 20017
1-866-899-5317
www.nopcas.com

Suicide Awareness Voices of Education
9001 E. Bloomington Fwy, Suite 150
Bloomington, MN 55420
(952) 946-7998
www.save.org

Suicide Prevention Action Network
1025 Vermont Avenue NW, Suite 1066
Washington, DC 20005
(202) 449-3600
www.spanusa.org

Substance Abuse

Alcoholics Anonymous
P.O. Box 459
New York, NY 10163
(212) 870-3400
www.aa.org

Narcotics Anonymous
P.O. Box 9999
Van Nuys, California 91409
(818) 773-9999
www.na.org

National Institute on Alcohol Abuse and Alcoholism
5635 Fishers Lane, MSC 9304
Bethesda, MD 20892-9304
(301) 443-3860
www.niaaa.nih.gov

National Institute on Drug Abuse
6001 Executive Boulevard, Room 5213
Bethesda, MD 20892-9561
(301) 443-1124
(240) 221-4007 (en Español)
www.nida.nih.gov

Substance Abuse and Mental Health Services Administration
1 Choke Cherry Road
Rockville, MD 20857
(240) 276-2000
www.samhsa.gov

Related Organizations

The following is a list of organizations that specialize in research or other areas in the mental health field.

American Psychiatric Association
1000 Wilson Boulevard, Suite 1825
Arlington, Va. 22209-3901
(703) 907-7300
www.psych.org

American Psychological Association
750 First Street, NE
Washington, DC 20002-4242
1- 800-374-2721
www.apa.org

Bazelon Center for Mental Health Law
1101 15th Street, NW, Suite 1212
Washington, DC 20005
(202) 467-5730
www.bazelon.org

Federation of Families for Children's Mental Health
9605 Medical Center Dr., Suite 280
Rockville, MD 20850
(240) 403-1901
www.ffcmh.org

National Institute of Mental Health
Public Information and Communications Branch
6001 Executive Blvd., Room 8184, MSC 9663
Bethesda, MD 20892-9663
1-866-615-6464
www.nimh.nih.gov

RESOURCES

New York University Child Study Center
577 First Avenue
New York, NY 10016
(212) 263-6622
www.aboutourkids.org

The Trevor Project
8950 West Olympic Blvd., Suite 197
Beverly Hills, CA 90211
(310) 271-8845
www.thetrevorproject.org

Suggested Readings

Abramson, John.
Overdosed America: The Broken Promise of American Medicine.
Harper Collins, 2004.

Griffith, Gail.
Will's Choice: A Suicidal Teen, A Desperate Mother, and a Chronicle of Recovery.
Harper Collins, 2005.

Jamison, Kay Redfield.
An Unquiet Mind: A Memoir of Moods and Madness.
Knopf, 1995.

Jamison, Kay Redfield.
Night Falls Fast: Understanding Suicide.
Random House, 1999.

Kadison, Richard. Digeronimo, Theresa Foy.
College of the Overwhelmed: The Campus Mental Health Crisis and What to do About it.
Jossey-Bass, 2004.

BehindHappyFaces.com

Koplewicz, Harold.
More Than Moody; Recognizing and Treating Adolescent Depression.
G.P. Putnam and Sons, 2002.

Levenkron, Steven.
Cutting: Understanding and Overcoming Self-Mutilation.
W.W. Norton and Company, 1998.

Simon, Lizzie.
Detour: My Bipolar Trip in 4-D.
Simon & Schuster, Inc., 2003.

Solomon, Andrew.
The Noonday Demon: An Atlas of Depression.
Simon & Schuster, Inc., 2001.

Weiner, Jessica.
Do I Look Fat in This?: Life Doesn't Begin Five Pounds from Now.
Simon & Schuster, Inc., 2005.

Weiner, Jessica.
A Very Hungry Girl: How I Filled Up On Life...and How You Can, Too!
Hay House, Inc., 2003.

Zailckas, Koren.
Smashed: Story of a Drunken Girlhood.
Viking, Penguin, 2006.

How Can I Get Involved?

The following organizations offer ways for you to get involved in the mental health movement either on your campus or in your community. If you would like to bring a speaker to your school, start a chapter to promote mental health awareness, host mental health weeks, walks, runs, or any other idea you may have, you can find all of the information you need from the organizations listed here!

National Mental Health Awareness Campaign
P.O. Box 491608
Los Angeles, CA 90049
www.nostigma.org

** Book a speaker like Ross Szabo and others, from the only mental health speakers' bureau in the country!

Active Minds
1875 Connecticut Ave, NW Suite 418
Washington, DC 20009
(202) 719-1177
www.activemindsoncampus.org

Develops and supports student-run mental health awareness, education, and advocacy groups on the college campus.

The BACCHUS Network™
P.O. Box 100430
Denver, CO 80250
(303) 871-0901
www.bacchusgamma.org

University and community-based network of over 32,000 student leaders and advisors who work with over eight million peers on more than 900 campuses throughout the world. Develops cutting-edge tools for campuses focusing on comprehensive health and safety initiatives.

Compeer Inc.
400 Andrews St., Suite 340
Rochester, NY 14604
1-800-836-0475
www.compeer.org

International non-profit organization helping adults and children overcome the effects of mental illness through the power of friendship. Volunteer-based programs and services, which serve as a complement to therapy, provide supportive friendships for people in mental-health care—helping them on their recovery journey.

CampusBlues.com/ReconnectingU
328 Monomoscoy Road
Mashpee, MA 02649
(508) 477-4002
www.campusblues.com
www.reconnectingu.com

CampusBlues.com is an innovative program designed to facilitate student awareness and use of campus counseling centers and other school support services. Looking to reduce the stigma associated with seeking help, this program makes it easier for students to do so. They can also recommend alternatives for students unable or unwilling to utilize school resources. By offering quality, accessible and affordable assistance services, ReconnectingU is dedicated to supporting the mental health and well being of individuals as they move through their personal transitions.

RESOURCES

Depression and Bipolar Support Alliance (DBSA)
730 N. Franklin Street, Suite 501
Chicago, IL 60610-7224
1-800-826 -3632
www.dbsalliance.org

The leading patient-directed national organization focusing on the most prevalent mental illnesses. DBSA fosters an environment of understanding by providing up-to-date, scientifically-based tools and information written in language the general public can understand, and works to ensure that people living with mood disorders are treated equitably.

Mental Health America (MHA)
2000 N. Beauregard Street, 6th Floor
Alexandria, Virginia 22311
(703) 684-7722
www.mentalhealthamerica.net

With more than 320 affiliates nationwide, MHA is the country's leading nonprofit dedicated to helping ALL people live mentally healthier lives.MHA represents a growing movement of Americans who promote mental wellness for the health and well-being of the nation—everyday and in times of crisis.

Mpower Concert Initiative
Musicians for Mental Health
c/o NMHA
2000 N. Beauregard St., 6th floor
Alexandria, VA 22311
800-969-6642
www.mpoweryouth.org

Sponsored by the National Mental Health Association (NMHA), mpower is a new youth awareness campaign to change

BehindHappyFaces.com

attitudes about mental health and fight the stigma facing the 1 in 5 youth with mental health problems. Working with a diverse coalition of artists, music industry executives, mental health advocates and youth leaders, mpower will utilize concert tie-ins, special events, media activities, PSAs, educational forums and web-based outreach to empower millions of young people to get informed...and take action.

mtvU and Jed Foundation College Mental Health Awareness Campaign
www.halfofus.com

Interactive website and campaign launched by mtvU and The Jed Foundation to raise awareness about the prevalence of mental health issues on campus, and connect students to appropriate resources where they can get help.

NAMI (National Alliance for the Mentally Ill)
NAMI on Campus
Colonial Place Three
2107 Wilson Blvd., Suite 300
Arlington, VA 22201-3042
(703) 524-7600
www.nami.org

NAMI is the nation's largest grassroots mental health organization dedicated to the eradication of mental illnesses and to the improvement of the quality of life of all whose lives are affected by these diseases. NAMI on Campus affiliates are student-run, student-led organizations providing mental health support, education, and advocacy in a campus setting. Their mission is to improve the lives of students who are directly or indirectly affected by mental illness, increase the awareness and mental health services on campus, and to eliminate the stigma facing students with mental illness.

RESOURCES

The Rita Project
1-866-775-RITA
www.ritaproject.org

A 501c3 non-profit organization devoted to using the arts to help survivors of suicide connect with the power of creation, and in doing so, foster transformation. A global movement to stop suicide...and to celebrate life.

Screening for Mental Health, Inc. (SMH)
One Washington Street, Suite 304
Wellesley Hills, MA 02481
(781) 239-0071
www.mentalhealthscreening.org

SMH first introduced the concept of large-scale mental health screenings with National Depression Screening Day in 1991. SMH programs now include both in-person and online programs for depression, bipolar disorder, generalized anxiety disorder, post-traumatic stress disorder, eating disorders, alcohol problems, and suicide prevention.

Substance Abuse and Mental Health Services Administration
www.whatadifference.samhsa.gov

Website for people living with mental illness—and their friends. You'll find tools to help in the recovery process, read real-life stories about support and recovery, and see how friends can make all the difference.

Suicide Prevention Action Network (SPAN USA)
1025 Vermont Avenue, NW, Suite 1066
Washington, DC 20005
Phone: (202) 449-3600
www.spanusa.org

BehindHappyFaces.com

The nation's only suicide prevention organization dedicated to leveraging grassroots support among suicide survivors (those who have lost a loved one to suicide) and others to advance public policies that help prevent suicide.

ENDNOTES

Chapter 1

1. Page 24. "In 2005, nearly half (47%) of college freshmen had an A average in high school, compared with 20% in 1970. And as students' grades improve, so do their material expectations for their lives. In 2005, 75% of college freshmen said their primary objective was 'being very well off financially,' while back in 1970, 79% of college freshmen wanted to 'develop a meaningful philosophy of life.'" **http://www.census.gov/Press-Release/ www/releases/archives/miscellaneous/007871.html**

2. Page 25. "The national divorce rate is close to 50%." **http://www. divorcereform.org/rates.html**

3. Page 27. "While the rates of people using marijuana, cocaine, heroine, and some other hard-core drugs have slightly declined, the use of crystal meth and prescription drugs maintained a high level of abuse." Substance Abuse and Mental Health Services Administration **http://www. drugabusestatistics.samhsa.gov/prescription/toc.htm**

4. Page 28. "Over 44% of college students report binge drinking" Kadison, Richard. Digeronimo, Theresa Foy. *College of the Overwhelmed: The Campus Mental Health Crisis and What to do About it.* San Francisco: Jossey-Bass, 2004.

5. Page 28. "and two-thirds of young people with a substance use disorder have a co-occurring mental health issue." 1999 Surgeon General's Report on Suicide and Mental Health **http://www.surgeongeneral.gov/library/ mentalhealth/toc.html**

ENDNOTES

6. Page 28. "80% of college students are sexually active." UCI Health Education Sexual Health Program **http://www.health.uci.edu/forms/ thegoodnews.pdf**

7. Page 28. 47% of high school students are sexually active. **http://www. kff.org/youthhivstds/upload/U-S-Teen-Sexual-Activity-Fact-Sheet.pdf**

8. Page 31-36. Descriptions of mental disorders from the National Institute of Mental Health.

9. Page 37. "Statistics show that a large majority of people who seek help can see improvement in their symptoms." 1999 Surgeon General's Report on Suicide and Mental Health **http://www.surgeongeneral.gov/library/ mentalhealth/toc.html**

10. Page 37. "Suicide is the third leading cause of death in people ages 15-24 and the second leading cause of death on college campuses." The Jed Foundation **http://www.jedfoundation.org/documents/YouthSuicide.pdf**

Chapter 2

1. Page 44. "66% of young people do not seek help for a mental disorder." National Comorbidity Survey Replication **http://www.hcp.med.harvard. edu/ncs/**

2. Page 51. "One out of 5 high school students and one out of 4 college students has mental disorder." National Institute of Mental Health **http:// www.nimh.nih.gov/healthinformation/statisticsmenu.cfm**

3. Page 61. "A recent study showed that 25% of people in our country feel they have no one they can confide in. 75% of respondents said they feel that they can confide in one person." American Sociological Review June 2006 **http://www.asanet.org/page.ww?section=Press&name=circle+of+friends**

Chapter 3

1. Page 79. "Over 57 million American adults are affected by one or more mental disorders each year." National Institute of Mental Health **http:// www.nimh.nih.gov/healthinformation/statisticsmenu.cfm**

2. Page 80. "Women twice as likely to experience depression, more likely to attempt taking their own lives, more likely to develop eating disorder." National Institute of Mental Health **http://www.nimh.nih.gov/publicat/numbers.cfm**

3. Page 80. "As many as 10 million women suffer from anorexia and bulimia. Approximately 25 million more suffer from binge eating disorder. Eating disorders are among the deadliest and most difficult mental disorders to treat." National Eating Disorders Association **http://www.nationaleatingdisorders.org/p.asp?WebPage_ID=286&Profile_ID=41138**

4. Page 80. "Women also are two times as likely to experience generalized anxiety disorder." 1999 Surgeon General's Report on Suicide and Mental Health **http://www.surgeongeneral.gov/library/mentalhealth/chapter4/sec2.html**

5. Page 80. "Women more likely to seek help." World Health Organization **http://www.who.int/mental_health/prevention/genderwomen/en/**

6. Page 80. "Women are more often victims of sexual abuse." Center for Disease Control **http://www.cdc.gov/ncipc/factsheets/svfacts.htm**

7. Page 80. "Women deal with more hormonal shifts." The Mayo Clinic **http://www.mayoclinic.com/health/depression/MH00035**

8. Page 84. "They are also more likely to suffer from anti-social behavior." Mayo Foundation for Education and Research **http://www.cnn.com/HEALTH/library/DS/00829.html**

9. Page 89. "A national survey revealed that out of the 596 licensed psychologists with active clinical practices who are members of the American Psychological Association, only 1% of the randomly selected sample identified themselves as Latino." Williams, S. and Kohout, J.L. *A survey of licensed practitioners of psychology: Activities, roles and services.* American Psychological Association, Washington D.C., 1999.

10. Page 89. "African Americans comprise less than 4% of mental health care providers nationally." **http://www.womensenews.org/article.cfm/dyn/aid/1392/context/archive**

ENDNOTES

11. Page 89. "In the late 1990's approximately 70 Asian American providers were available for every 100,000 Asian Americans in the U.S." 1999 Surgeon General's Report on Suicide and Mental Health **http://mentalhealth. samhsa.gov/cre/ch5_availability.asp**

12. Page 92. "Affluent suburban adolescents have been shown to be at greater risk for depression and drug use than are both middle-class and lower-class samples of young people." **http://findarticles.com/p/articles/ mi_m2248/is_158_40/ai_n14815096/pg_1**

Chapter 4

1. Page 107. "The counselor to student ratio is still 1 to 1,697 and some smaller schools have better ratios." National Survey of Counseling Center Directors 2006 "Alternative Treatments" box: SAMHSA's National Mental Health Information Center **http://www.iacsinc.org/National%20Survey%2 0for%20Counseling%20Center%20Directors%20Results%20-%20Final.pdf**

2. Page 116. "Alternative treatments box" **http://mentalhealth.samhsa. gov/publications/allpubs/ken98-0044/default.asp**

Chapter 5

1. Page 150. Information for this sidebar on what to say to your parents from The Jed Foundation. Permission for use granted by Program Director Joanna Locke.

2. Page 153. "If someone in your family has a diagnosable mental disorder you have a greater chance of developing the disorder." National Mental Health Awareness Campaign **http://www.nostigma.org/students_faqs. php?faq=07**

3. Page 160. "Suicide is second leading cause of death on college campuses." Haas, A. P. (2004) *Identifying and Treating Students at Risk for Suicide: The AFSP College Screening Project:* Presentation from the October 2004 SPRC Discussion Series.

4. Page 160. "In 2004, over 32,000 people took their own life." National Institute of Mental Health **http://www.nimh.nih.gov/publicat/numbers. cfm#Suicide**

5. Page 162. Sidebar Family that eats together stays together American Academy of Pediatrics **http://parenting247.org/article.cfm?ContentID=5 97&strategy=2&AgeGroup=4**

Chapter 6

1. Page 181. Information for this sidebar on "warning signs" from The Jed Foundation. Permission for use granted by Program Director Dr. Joanna Locke.

2. Page 188-189. Information for this sidebar on a friend who is suicidal from The Jed Foundation. Permission granted by Program Director Dr. Joanna Locke.

Chapter 7

1. Page 211. "Ninety percent of people who take their own lives have a co-occurring mental disorder." National Mental Health Association **http:// www1.nmha.org/shcr/community_based/costoffset.pdf**

Song/Film Credits

Songs

Page 21. Jagger, Mick and Keith Richards. "Mother's Little Helper." Lyrics. Rec. Dec 3-8 1965. *Aftermath*. Decca/ABKCO, 1966. © ABKCO Music, Inc.

Page 41. Thomas, Rob. "Unwell." Lyrics. Rec. 2002. *More Than You Think You Are*. Atlantic Records, 2003. © EMI Music Publishing.

Page 99. Nalick, Anna. "Breathe (2am)." Lyrics. *Wreck of the Day*. Columbia, 2005. © Annibonna Music.

Page 163. King, Joe and Isaac Slade. "How to Save a Life." Rec. 2004-2005. *How to Save a Life*. Epic Records, 2006. © Aaron Edwards Publishing, EMI/ April Music, Inc.

Page 191. Lightbody, Gary. "Chasing Cars." Lyrics. Rec 2005. *Eyes Open*. Interscope Records, 2006. © Songs of Windswept Pacific.

Films

Page 135. *Little Miss Sunshine*. Dir. Jonathan Dayton, Valerie Faris. Wrt. Michael Arndt. Dist. Fox Searchlight Pictures, © 2006.

ACKNOWLEDGMENTS

Ross Szabo

I could not have written this book, or done any of the traveling, work, or speaking that I have done over the past five years, without the love and support of my beautiful Heidi. Thank you so much, Baby—for putting up with everything in the most amazing and patient ways that you *always* do. You truly do make every day of my life better. I love you very much, and I'll be home soon.

I would like to thank Gail Kamer Lieberfarb for so many things, but mostly for recognizing the importance of speaking to young people about these issues, and for doing everything that she could in order to help *me* continue to do that. My thanks to Howard Goldman for his invaluable advice, perception, understanding and friendship—and for taking the time to review each chapter of this book as it was written. Thanks also to the rest of the board of the National Mental Health Awareness Campaign.

Special thanks go out to Melanie, whose amazing and emotional writing lifted this book to another level; my agent Bob Silverstein, for taking on this book; our publisher Jeff Stern, for his incredible foresight, friendship and enduring belief in this project; marketing/editorial director Lori Radcliff, for her thoughtful attention to detail and patience with our pressing deadlines; and finally to Adrianna, Josh and the rest of our Bonus Books team. We also thank Bonus for their high standards and artistic vision for this project—and bringing together the talents of designers Emily Brackett and Candice Woo, and photographer extraordinaire Cindy Gold (thanks for a perfect "Zoolander!")

I must also recognize the rest of our dedicated editorial team: Jennifer Repo, who helped us to assemble the first drafts of the manuscript; Sarah Thomson, our amazing content editor, whose vision and sensibility helped to make this book what it is; and finally, Marc Aronson—whose invaluable advice and support helped us at a crucial point to refine our collective vision for this book.

Special thanks to Shawn Sachs, Jay Strell, Kate Ottenberg and the team at Sunshine, Sachs & Associates for their boundless creativity, enthusiasm and persistence in helping to spread the word about this project.

I never would have had the chance to speak even one time, if not for one of the finest educators in the country, Bob Bryant. Thanks, Bob, for looking into that angry 17-year-old's eyes...and believing in him. (And if anyone is ever in PA's Lehigh Valley, be sure to check out the cool sounds of the Bryant Brothers Blues Brew!)

My best friends and their wives—in no specific order: Dave Serensits, Mark Sherman, Brent Fehnel and Shane Strike. Thanks for being there for me through all of this—you all mean so very much to me. Other peeps who have been there: my cousins Kevin, Lisa, Tony, and Macey Martin; more friends: Marc Adelman (get excited!), Mike Fleming, Alison Malmon,

Laura Evans, Laura Newhard, Robert Lang, Erin Weed and T.J. Sullivan; and every (current and former) employee of CAMPUSPEAK.

I would also like to thank *every* student, teacher, counselor, mom, dad, principal—and everyone else along the way (you know who you are!) who has thanked me for speaking, wished me well, hugged me, or shared their thoughts. Your words and letters continue to drive me forward, helping me to further understand the true importance of this message.

Last, and certainly not least, *my family.* My grandparents, aunts, uncles, and cousins—and most importantly, my amazing and wonderful parents, Paul and Fran. I am only now realizing just *how* appreciative I should have been to have parents like you. Thank you for continuing to define what your own lives should be, and not giving in to what others think. Thanks to my two brothers (and best friends) Thad and Vance, and my sister-in-law Micki. Thad, thank you especially for providing the positive example that gave me hope and understanding for this disorder, and for being there for me. Vance, you have the biggest heart in the world—I am lucky to have someone like you to care so much. I want to thank ALL of you for standing by me, and for being the wonderful people you are to bring this family back together, and for keeping us strong. *I love you all—very much.*

Melanie Hall

Behind Happy Faces would not exist without the support of so many extraordinary people. First, I want to echo Ross' thanks to our publisher Jeff Stern—as well as Lori Radcliff, our amazing editors, and all the folks at Bonus Books—for their commitment, vision and tenacity, and for believing so strongly in this project.

I would also like to personally thank Bob Silverstein for helping us to find the right home for our book.

I am so grateful to Jane Semel, my dear friend and mentor. You will never know how much your friendship—and our work together—has meant to me. Thank you for starting me on my path. I will always be deeply grateful for my time at iJane, and the opportunity you gave me to learn and hone both my creative skills and my voice as a writer.

Thank you to Gail Lieberfarb for introducing me to Ross and for befriending me in such a truly lovely way.

Special thanks to my dear friends and colleagues for providing insight, wisdom, laughter and ample procrastination fodder: Dana and Gary Slavett, Brooke Burns, Marshall Herskovitz, Stacy Erich, Jennifer Hughes, Carol Allen, Mary Lee Malcolm, Kimberlee Acquaro-Landesman, April Beyer, Lisa Cirincione, Carol Dietrich, Gabi Bigai, Eric Weissler, Sam Brown, Steve Serpas and Bill Partridge.

To my wonderful friends at Demand Media: Joe Perez, Richard Rosenblatt, Shawn Colo, Quinn Daly, Wadooah Wali, Mel Tang, Lori Dreishmeier, Shama Shamsudeen, Jeff Quandt, and Christine Andreocci. Thank you so much for supporting me as I attempted to balance a full-time job with a break-neck editing schedule! I will always be grateful for my time with you guys.

I must extend my heartfelt thanks to my family: Harvey, Lynne, Allison, Caroline, Eli, Guy and Kai. Thank you for your love, inspiration and kindness; for always taking my call (no matter the time of day—or night); and for always filling the cup so that it's half *full!* When it comes to my family, I truly won the lottery. I love you all very, very much. Moop on.

Finally, and most of all, I want to thank Ross Szabo. Ross, your dedication to helping others and allowing yourself to be an example is a true inspiration! Thank you for your patience, insight, understanding, humor, for keeping us on schedule, for your many text messages—and for asking me to partner with you on this special project. It has been an incredible opportunity, and one that I will always cherish.

ABOUT THE AUTHORS

ROSS SZABO is the Director of Youth Outreach for the National Mental Health Awareness Campaign (NMHAC) and a speaker for CAMPUSPEAK, Inc. Also the youngest speaker on mental health issues in the U.S., he has addressed over 500,000 students, parents, teachers and counselors in the last five years.

Szabo confronted the stigma of mental illness at an early age. A popular student leader and athlete, he was diagnosed with bipolar disorder at age 16. In his senior year of high school he was hospitalized for wanting to take his own life, and soon after his release, experienced the social isolation of the disease. His college years were also filled with emotional setbacks, as he was later forced to take a medical leave of absence from American University and was hospitalized again due to a relapse. Szabo returned to college in the fall of 2000, and began to use his broad understanding of mental health to educate others. After graduating cum laude with a Bachelor's of Arts degree in psychology from American University in 2002, he set out on a full-time mission to speak out about mental health issues—in an effort to reach young people who are struggling to deal with their problems, and to eradicate needless stereotypes.

Szabo's dynamic, relatable presentations and inspiring personal account of his experiences with mental illness have made him one of the top speakers on the college circuit—leading him to be named "Best Male Performer" by CAMPUS ACTIVITIES Magazine in early 2007. A regular speaker at national mental health conferences, Szabo has participated in major media events in recent years with the likes of NMHAC's Tipper Gore and former Surgeon General Dr. David Satcher. One of his popular high school presentations was turned into a regional PBS program entitled, "What's On Your Mind?" for WNED-TV (Buffalo/Toronto). Szabo has been interviewed about teen and young adult mental health by national publications including *PARADE* and *SEVENTEEN* magazines and major network and cable news outlets including CNN, CBS and MTV. He continues to develop educational middle school, high school and college programs while speaking to nearly 100,000 people each year. Szabo resides in Los Angeles, CA.

MELANIE HALL has long been a pioneer of social media networks for young people. While serving as president of ijane inc., a non-profit production company promoting public health issues, Hall created, produced and directed the "Face The Issue" Public Service Announcement (PSA) campaign. Addressing the mental health issues facing young adults, the campaign included seven animated PSAs featuring celebrity narrators including Halle Berry, Nicole Kidman, Jennifer Lopez, Sarah Jessica Parker and others, and the website **facetheissue.com.** The PSAs received recognition by The Prism Awards and various network news outlets including CNN, and *The New York Times* claimed the campaign was "a model for what future communications with young people will look like."

While at ijane, Hall also created the animated interactive application for UCLA's "Internet Treatment Delivery of Parent-Adolescent Conflict Training for Families with an ADHD Teen: A Feasibility Study." The animated shorts were the cornerstone of the study, funded by The Oppenheimer Foundation. The project examined the feasibility of Internet delivery of a Parent-Adolescent Conflict Training (PACT) program to families with an ADHD teen.

Before co-founding ijane with Jane Semel, Hall wrote and produced the award-winning *The Spot*, the first original episodic series to be broadcast online. As a result, America Online asked her to write and produce *Entertainment Asylum*, AOL's entertainment initiative. Simultaneously, iXL, a global strategic marketing company for Fortune 500 companies, recruited Hall to conceive and produce strategies for global brands such as *FritoLay, Doritos, Yahoo!, Excite, Lycos, WebMD* and Warner Bros. among others, in order to establish a competitive online presence.

A native of New Orleans, Louisiana, Hall currently resides in Los Angeles, California, where she spends much of her spare time cycling, skiing, and enjoying many other outdoor sports.

INDEX

INDEX

INDEX

I

impulsive behavior, 34–35, 88, 181
insomnia
  see sleep and sleep deprivation
insurance, 92–93, 106–107, 120, 161

J

The Jed Foundation, 181, 188–89, 231, 239

K

Kadison, Richard, 131–33
Kirsten Brooks Hope center, 231
Knowledge Exchange Network, 227
krumping, 94–95

L

legal rights, 106–8
Levenkron, Steven, 68
LGBTQ (Lesbian, Gay, Bisexual, Transgender and Questioning), 95–97
lifestyle changes, 116–19, 148
loneliness, 36, 43, 75, 174
loss of friends, 77, 176–78
  see also breakups
love
  see romantic relationships

M

maintenance, 127–31
manic depression
  see bipolar disorder
media images, 49, 79
medical insurance, 92–93
medications (treatment), 38, 39, 82, 91, 93, 102, 105, 111–16, 120–121, 124, 155
men, 39, 78, 80, 83–88, 168
mental disorders
  about, 21–39
  common (and symptoms of), 31-36
  and families, 136–62
  and friends, 163–89
  genetic components, 153
  media images of, 49
  and men, 39, 78, 80, 83–88, 100, 168
  personal stories, 21–23, 62, 122–23
  and physical health, 110, 121, 187, 210
  and poverty and wealth, 79, 90–95
  and race, 73–98
  resources, 227–41
  and romantic relationships, 191–218
  seeking help, 103–33
  stereotypes of, 78–79

stigma, 37, 44–49, 96, 219–21, 236, 237, 239, 240, 255
  and women, 39, 68, 79–82, 84, 168
  see also education; specific disorders
mental health
  introduction to, xvii–xix
    (Introduction), 23–24
  taking charge of your, 23, 31, 37, 50, 110, 103–133, 158, 215–216, 219–221
  see also mental disorders
Mental Health America, 238
minorities, 88–90
monitoring medications, 112
mood swings, 41, 181
Mpower Concert Initiative, 238–39
mtvU, 181, 239
music, 67, 116, 148, 239
Musicians for Mental Health, 239

N

Narcotics Anonymous, 232
National Alliance for Research on Schizophrenia and Depression, 230
National Alliance for the Mentally Ill, 239
National Eating Disorders Association, 230
National Hopeline Network, 228
National Institute of Mental Health, 233
National Institute on Alcohol Abuse and Alcoholism, 232
National Institute on Drug Abuse, 232
National Mental Health Awareness Campaign, 236, 255–56
National Organization for People of Color Against Suicide, 231
National Suicide Prevention Hotline, 228
New York University Child Study Center, 233
normalcy, 51–52, 130

O

obsessive-compulsive disorder, 32, 63, 93

P

pain
  and destructive friendships, 167–70, 187
  emotional, 28, 56, 69, 73, 84–85, 151, 195–96
  physical, 67–68, 85
panic, 32, 51
parents
  divorce, 23, 25, 30, 27, 59, 63, 69, 105, 110, 146, 148, 215

INDEX